THE ULTIMATE GASTRIC SLEEVE BARIATRIC COOKBOOK

Easy and nutritious bariatric friendly recipes For Healthy Stomach Recovery and Weight Loss After Surgery

Dr. Mary D. Cook

Text Copyright© 2024 by Dr. Mary D. Cook

All rights reserved worldwide No part of this publication may be republished in any form or by any means, including photocopying, scanning or otherwise without prior written permission to the copyright holder.

This book contains nonfictional content. The views expressed are those of the author and do not necessarily represent those of the publisher. In addition, the publisher declaims any responsibility for them.

TABLE OF CONTENTS

INTRODUCTION

Greetings, dear readers. I am Dr. Mary D. Cook, a seasoned nutritionist with a passion for guiding individuals towards optimal health and wellness. With a wealth of experience in the field, I am thrilled to present to you the "GASTRIC SLEEVE BARIATRIC COOKBOOK: Easy and nutritious bariatric-friendly recipes for Healthy Stomach Recovery and Weight Loss After Surgery."

In the realm of nutrition, I have witnessed firsthand the transformative power of a well-crafted diet, especially in the context of post-surgery recovery. Allow me to share a poignant real-life story that underscores the impact of tailored nutrition on the healing journey.

A few years ago, my dear in-law underwent gastric sleeve surgery, a decision not made lightly but driven by a fervent desire for a healthier and more fulfilling life. It was during this crucial recovery phase that I had the privilege of applying my nutritional expertise to facilitate her healing process.

Crafting a diet plan tailored to her specific needs and post-surgery requirements, we embarked on a journey of nourishment and rejuvenation. The recipes that form the core of this cookbook were, in part, inspired by this transformative experience. Witnessing the positive effects of a carefully curated diet plan on her overall well-being was nothing short of remarkable.

As the weeks unfolded, the results were evident — not only in the rapid recovery of her physical health but also in the remarkable weight loss that ensued. The journey was not without its challenges, but the power of nutrition to facilitate healing became an undeniable truth. It was a testament to the potential for transformation that lies within the choices we make at the dining table.

This cookbook, born from a genuine desire to share the knowledge and experiences that have shaped my career, is a tribute to the countless individuals navigating the post-surgery landscape. It is a guide, a companion, and a source of inspiration as you embark on your own journey towards health and well-being.

Join me as we explore the world of bariatric-friendly recipes designed not just for sustenance but for the joy of eating well. Let this cookbook be a beacon of hope, a roadmap to recovery, and a celebration of the incredible potential that lies within each nourishing bite.

To your health and happiness,

{Dr. Mary D. Cook}

Understanding Gastric Sleeve Surgery

Gastric sleeve surgery, also known as sleeve gastrectomy, is a surgical weight-loss procedure designed to assist individuals in achieving significant and sustained weight loss. This surgery involves the removal of a large portion of the stomach, resulting in a sleeve-shaped organ that is roughly the size of a banana.

The procedure begins with the surgeon making small incisions in the abdomen. Subsequently, a laparoscope, a small tube with a camera attached, is inserted to provide a visual guide for the surgery. The surgeon then carefully removes approximately 75-80% of the stomach, leaving behind the sleeve-like structure.

The primary objective of gastric sleeve surgery is twofold. Firstly, by reducing the size of the stomach, the surgery restricts the amount of food that can be consumed at any given time, leading to a feeling of fullness with smaller meals. This helps in controlling portion sizes and curbing excessive calorie intake.

Secondly, the surgery also involves the removal of the part of the stomach that produces the hunger-stimulating hormone ghrelin.

With reduced ghrelin levels, patients often experience a diminished appetite, contributing to long-term weight loss success.

Gastric sleeve surgery is considered a relatively straightforward and effective bariatric procedure, providing both restrictive and hormonal benefits. It is particularly suitable for individuals with obesity-related health issues, aiming not only to facilitate weight loss but also to improve or resolve associated conditions such as type 2 diabetes, high blood pressure, and sleep apnea.

As with any surgical procedure, gastric sleeve surgery requires careful consideration and consultation with healthcare professionals. It is essential for individuals considering this surgery to be well-informed about the potential risks, benefits, and lifestyle changes that accompany the post-operative period. Patients typically undergo thorough pre-operative evaluations to ensure they are suitable candidates for the surgery and are committed to adopting the necessary lifestyle changes for long-term success.

Importance of Nutrition Post-Surgery

The importance of nutrition for individuals undergoing gastric sleeve surgery is paramount, playing a crucial role in both the short-term recovery and the long-term success of the procedure. Here are key aspects that highlight the significance of nutrition in the context of gastric sleeve surgery:

1. Facilitating Healing and Recovery:

After gastric sleeve surgery, the body undergoes a significant transformation as a portion of the stomach is removed. Adequate nutrition is essential to support the healing process, ensuring that the body receives the necessary nutrients for tissue repair and recovery.

2. Meeting Nutrient Requirements:

The surgery alters the digestive system, impacting the body's ability to absorb certain nutrients efficiently. It becomes imperative to follow a nutrition plan that addresses the specific needs of post-surgery life. This includes prioritizing protein, vitamins, and minerals to prevent deficiencies and promote overall health.

3. Managing Weight Loss:

Nutrition is a cornerstone of successful weight loss after gastric sleeve surgery. The procedure restricts the stomach's capacity, leading to smaller meal sizes. A well-balanced and nutrient-dense diet helps individuals achieve weight loss goals while ensuring they receive the necessary energy and nutrients for daily functioning.

4. Preventing Complications:

Proper nutrition is vital in minimizing the risk of complications post-surgery. This includes avoiding nutritional deficiencies, which could lead to issues such as anemia or osteoporosis. Nutrient-rich foods and, if necessary, supplements are often prescribed to mitigate these risks.

5. Building Healthy Eating Habits:

Gastric sleeve surgery necessitates a shift in eating habits. Adopting a nutritious diet helps individuals establish and maintain healthy eating patterns. Learning to make nutrient-dense food choices and practicing portion control are essential components of sustainable weight management.

6. Enhancing Overall Well-Being:

Beyond weight loss, a well-rounded nutrition plan contributes to overall well-being. It can improve energy levels, mood, and mental clarity. Additionally, proper nutrition supports the body's immune function, reducing the likelihood of illness and promoting a healthier, more active lifestyle.

7. Supporting Lifestyle Changes:

Nutrition is integral to the broader lifestyle changes required for long-term success. Educating individuals on making healthier food choices, developing mindful eating habits, and incorporating regular physical activity are crucial components of post-surgery care.

In essence, the importance of nutrition for gastric sleeve surgery extends far beyond weight loss. It is a fundamental aspect of comprehensive care, ensuring that individuals not only achieve their desired weight goals but also experience improved health and quality of life in the aftermath of this transformative surgery.

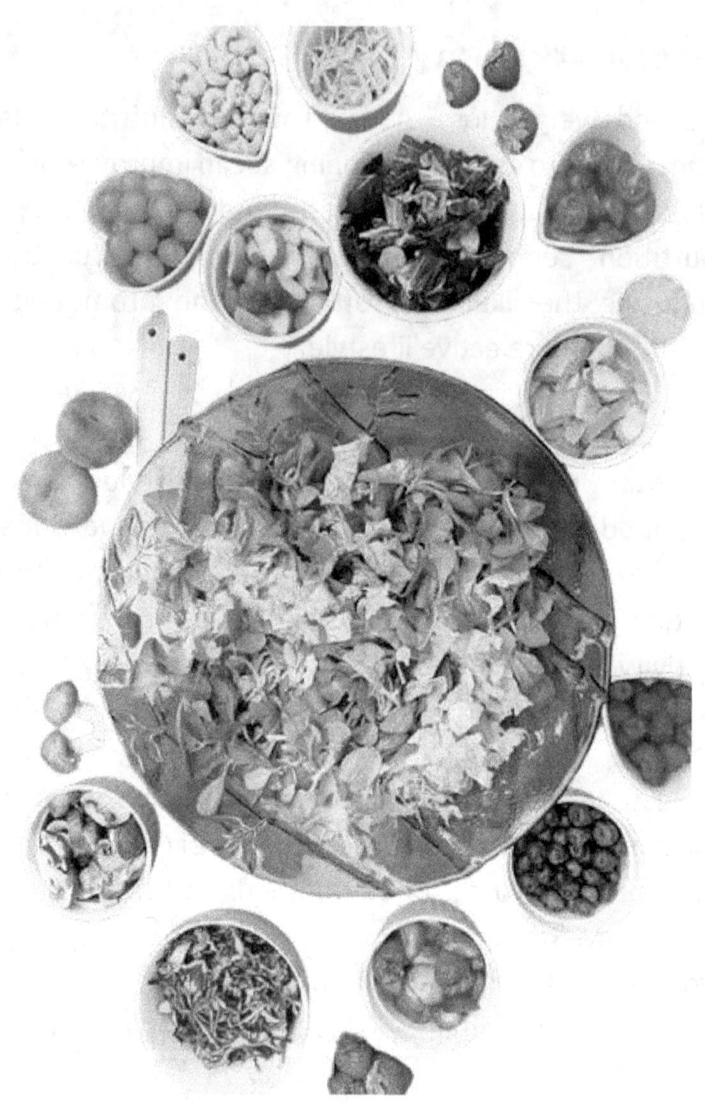

CHAPTER 1:

The Basics of Gastric Sleeve Nutrition

Nutrient Requirements After Surgery:

Following gastric sleeve surgery, the body undergoes a significant transformation that necessitates a focused approach to nutrient intake. Understanding and meeting these altered nutrient requirements is crucial for supporting the healing process, preventing deficiencies, and ensuring optimal health post-surgery.

1. Protein Emphasis:

Protein takes center stage in post-gastric sleeve nutrition. Adequate protein intake becomes essential for promoting tissue repair, maintaining muscle mass, and supporting overall recovery. Lean sources of protein, such as poultry, fish, eggs, and plant-based options, are emphasized to meet these heightened needs.

2. Vitamin and Mineral Considerations:

The surgery can impact the body's ability to absorb certain vitamins and minerals efficiently.

Therefore, attention is directed towards foods rich in nutrients like iron, calcium, vitamin B12, and vitamin D. Additionally, supplementation may be recommended to address potential deficiencies and promote long-term health.

3. Hydration Importance:

Staying hydrated is paramount in the post-surgery phase. Adequate water intake aids in digestion, nutrient absorption, and overall well-being. However, the reduced stomach size necessitates a mindful approach to fluid consumption, encouraging sips throughout the day to prevent dehydration while avoiding excessive drinking during meals.

4 .Balancing Carbohydrates and Fats:

Carbohydrates and fats are also integral components of a balanced diet. Emphasis is placed on choosing complex carbohydrates, such as whole grains and vegetables, to provide sustained energy. Healthy fats, sourced from avocados, nuts, and olive oil, contribute to satiety and support nutrient absorption.

5. Monitoring Sugar and Fiber Intake:

Post-surgery, sensitivity to certain foods, particularly those high in sugar, may increase.

Monitoring sugar intake is crucial for preventing discomfort and supporting weight loss.

Simultaneously, incorporating fiber-rich foods aids in digestion and helps individuals feel full with smaller portions.

Understanding these post-surgery nutrient requirements forms the basis for informed dietary choices. By tailoring the diet to meet these specific needs, individuals can enhance the healing process, minimize potential complications, and pave the way for sustained weight loss and overall well-being on their journey after gastric sleeve surgery. Regular consultations with healthcare professionals are recommended to ensure individualized and optimal nutrient intake.

Portion Control and Eating Habits:

In the post-gastric sleeve surgery phase, mastering portion control and cultivating mindful eating habits are pivotal for achieving optimal health, supporting weight loss, and adapting to the changes in stomach capacity.

1. Recognizing Satiety Cues:

With a reduced stomach size, it's essential to pay close attention to the body's satiety signals. This involves learning to recognize feelings of fullness and satisfaction during meals, preventing overeating. Slowing down the pace of eating and savoring each bite can enhance awareness of these cues, promoting a healthier relationship with food.

2. Smaller, Frequent Meals:

Instead of consuming large meals, the focus shifts towards smaller, more frequent meals throughout the day. This approach helps manage hunger, prevents discomfort, and optimizes nutrient absorption. Dividing daily caloric intake into several mini-meals supports a steady release of energy and facilitates adherence to recommended dietary guidelines.

3. Mindful Eating Practices:

Mindful eating involves being present and fully engaged during meals. Techniques such as chewing food thoroughly, putting down utensils between bites, and eliminating distractions (like screens) during meals contribute to a more conscious eating experience. This mindfulness fosters an appreciation for the flavors and textures of food while promoting better digestion.

4. Avoiding Grazing and Snacking Pitfalls:

While small, frequent meals are encouraged, grazing and continuous snacking are discouraged. Snacking between meals can contribute to excess calorie consumption. Establishing structured eating times and incorporating nutrient-dense snacks when needed helps strike a balance between satiety and weight management.

5. Hydration Timing:

Hydration is essential, but the timing of fluid intake is crucial to avoid diluting stomach acids during meals. Drinking fluids between meals rather than with food helps maintain stomach acidity for effective digestion. Sipping water throughout the day is encouraged, with a focus on hydration between meals rather than during.

6. Planning and Preparing Meals:

Effective portion control begins with planning and preparing meals thoughtfully. This involves measuring ingredients, using smaller plates, and being mindful of portion sizes. Planning meals in advance enables individuals to create balanced and satisfying dishes that align with their nutritional goals.

Mastering portion control and cultivating mindful eating habits contribute not only to successful weight management but also to an improved relationship with food. By incorporating these practices into daily life, individuals can navigate the post-surgery period with confidence, optimizing the benefits of gastric sleeve surgery and promoting long-term health and well-being. Regular consultations with healthcare professionals and nutritionists are recommended to tailor these principles to individual needs.

CHAPTER 2:

Preparing Your Kitchen for Success

Stocking Bariatric-Friendly Ingredients

Creating a kitchen that supports your post-gastric sleeve surgery journey begins with thoughtfully stocking bariatric-friendly ingredients. These carefully selected items form the foundation for preparing nutritious, satisfying meals that align with the specific needs of individuals who have undergone this transformative procedure.

1. Lean Proteins:

Prioritize the inclusion of lean protein sources in your kitchen. Opt for items such as skinless poultry, lean cuts of beef or pork, fish, eggs, and plant-based proteins like tofu and legumes. These protein sources are essential for muscle maintenance, tissue repair, and sustaining a feeling of fullness.

2. Variety of Vegetables:

Fill your refrigerator and pantry with a colorful array of vegetables.

Fresh, frozen, or canned vegetables without added sugars or sauces are excellent choices. These veggies provide essential vitamins, minerals, and fiber, contributing to overall health and aiding in digestion.

3. Whole Grains:

Incorporate whole grains into your pantry staples. Items like quinoa, brown rice, oats, and whole wheat products add complex carbohydrates and fiber to your diet. Whole grains release energy gradually, promoting sustained fullness and helping manage blood sugar levels.

4. Healthy Fats:

Include sources of healthy fats in your kitchen, such as avocados, nuts, seeds, and olive oil. These fats contribute to satiety, support the absorption of fat-soluble vitamins, and enhance the flavor and texture of your meals.

5. Low-Sugar Fruits:

Choose low-sugar fruits for added sweetness without excessive sugar intake. Berries, melons, and citrus fruits are excellent options. Limiting high-sugar fruits helps manage calorie intake and supports weight management goals.

6. Dairy or Dairy Alternatives:

Depending on individual tolerances, stock up on dairy or dairy alternatives that are low in fat and sugar. Options like Greek yogurt, low-fat cheese, and fortified plant-based milks contribute calcium and protein to your diet.

7. Clear Soups and Broths:

Keep clear soups and broths on hand as they provide hydration and can be a nourishing addition to your meals. Opt for low-sodium options to control your salt intake.

8. Herbs and Spices:

Enhance the flavor of your dishes with a variety of herbs and spices. This allows you to reduce reliance on salt or high-calorie sauces, making your meals both tasty and health-conscious.

9. Hydration Choices:

Ensure you have hydration options readily available. This includes water, herbal teas, and other low-calorie beverages. Staying adequately hydrated is crucial for digestion and overall well-being.

10. Protein Supplements (if recommended):

Depending on individual requirements and dietary habits, consider having protein supplements, such as shakes or powders, on hand. These can serve as convenient options to meet protein goals when whole food sources may be challenging.

By strategically stocking your kitchen with these bariatric-friendly ingredients, you set the stage for creating diverse, flavorful, and nutritionally balanced meals that align with your post-surgery dietary guidelines. Regularly reassessing and replenishing these staples ensures that your kitchen remains a supportive environment for your health and wellness journey.

Essential Cooking Tools

Equipping your kitchen with the right tools is essential for creating bariatric-friendly meals that are easy to prepare, nutritious, and enjoyable. Here's a guide to the essential cooking tools that will streamline your culinary experience post-gastric sleeve surgery:

1. Quality Chef's Knife:

Invest in a high-quality chef's knife for precision and ease in chopping, slicing, and dicing. A sharp knife makes meal preparation more efficient and enjoyable.

2. Cutting Boards:

Have durable, easy-to-clean cutting boards to create a hygienic and practical workspace. Consider using color-coded boards for different food groups to prevent cross-contamination.

3. Measuring Cups and Spoons:

Accurate portioning is crucial, and measuring cups and spoons help ensure precision in ingredient quantities, especially when dealing with limited portion sizes post-surgery.

4. Food Scale:

A digital food scale provides an accurate way to measure ingredients by weight, supporting portion control and adherence to dietary guidelines.

5. Non-Stick Cookware:

Opt for non-stick pans and pots to reduce the need for excessive oil when cooking. This helps in preparing meals that are lower in fat while preventing food from sticking to the cookware.

6. Steamer Basket:

A steamer basket is a versatile tool for cooking vegetables, proteins, and grains without the need for added fats. Steaming preserves nutrients and enhances the natural flavors of foods.

7. Blender or Food Processor:

A blender or food processor is invaluable for creating smoothies, purees, and soups. These appliances enable you to incorporate a variety of nutrient-dense ingredients into easily digestible and flavorful dishes.

8. Baking Sheets and Pans:

Have a selection of baking sheets and pans for roasting vegetables, lean proteins, and creating balanced, oven-baked meals. This cooking method enhances flavor without excessive use of oils.

9. Silicone Utensils:

Silicone utensils are gentle on non-stick surfaces and make stirring, flipping, and serving meals easier. They are heat-resistant and durable, ensuring longevity in your kitchen.

10. Strainer or Colander:

A strainer or colander is essential for draining excess liquids from foods like vegetables or cooked grains, contributing to the creation of balanced and satisfying dishes.

11. Instant-Read Thermometer:

Ensure proteins are cooked to a safe temperature with an Instant-read thermometer. This tool promotes food safety and helps prevent overcooking.

12. Food Storage Containers:

Invest in a variety of sizes of food storage containers for portioning and storing leftovers. This promotes organization and makes meal planning and preparation more efficient.

13. Slow Cooker or Instant Pot:

These versatile appliances are excellent for preparing nutritious, one-pot meals with minimal effort. They are especially convenient for individuals with a busy lifestyle.

By assembling these essential cooking tools, you create a kitchen environment that supports your post-surgery dietary goals. These tools not only enhance the efficiency of meal preparation but also contribute to the enjoyment of the cooking process. Regularly maintaining and organizing your kitchen tools ensures a smooth and enjoyable cooking experience on your health and wellness journey.

Meal Planning Tips

Effective meal planning is a cornerstone of successful post-gastric sleeve surgery nutrition. It ensures that your dietary choices align with your health goals, providing a foundation for balanced, nutritious, and enjoyable eating. Here are essential tips to streamline your meal planning process:

1. Set Realistic Goals:

Establish achievable and realistic dietary goals. Consider factors such as your nutritional requirements, weight loss objectives, and lifestyle. Realistic goals set the stage for sustainable changes.

2. Prioritize Protein:

Make protein a focal point in your meal planning. Incorporate lean protein sources like poultry, fish, tofu, and legumes into each meal to support muscle maintenance and satiety.

3. Include a Variety of Vegetables:

Diversify your vegetable intake to ensure a broad spectrum of nutrients. Experiment with different colors, textures, and cooking methods to keep your meals interesting and nutritionally rich.

4. Incorporate Whole Grains:

Choose whole grains for sustained energy and added fiber. Options like quinoa, brown rice, and oats contribute essential nutrients while promoting satiety.

5. Embrace Healthy Fats:

Integrate sources of healthy fats, such as avocados, nuts, and olive oil, into your meals. These fats support nutrient absorption and add flavor to your dishes.

6. Mindful Portioning:

Practice portion control to align with your surgery's effects on stomach capacity. Use measuring tools, smaller plates, and mindful eating practices to prevent overeating.

7. Plan Balanced Meals:

Aim for balanced meals that include a combination of protein, vegetables, whole grains, and healthy fats. This approach maximizes nutritional intake and supports overall well-being.

8. Hydration Awareness:

Prioritize hydration by incorporating water-rich foods and scheduling regular water breaks between meals. Staying adequately hydrated supports digestion and overall health.

9. Prepare Snacks Wisely:

Plan for nutritious snacks to curb hunger between meals. Opt for options like Greek yogurt, nuts, or cut vegetables to maintain energy levels without compromising on nutritional value.

10. Batch Cooking and Meal Prep:

Save time by batch cooking and meal prepping. Prepare larger quantities of staple items and portion them into containers for quick and convenient access throughout the week.

11. Experiment with Recipes:

Keep your meals exciting by experimenting with new recipes.

Discovering innovative ways to prepare familiar ingredients adds variety to your diet and keeps your palate engaged.

12. Flexibility and Adaptability:

Be flexible with your meal plans. Life is dynamic, and unexpected events may arise. Having a flexible approach allows you to adapt without feeling stressed or defeated.

13. Record and Reflect:

Keep a food diary to track your meals and reflect on how different foods make you feel. This self-awareness can aid in refining your meal plans and identifying patterns that support your well-being.

By incorporating these meal planning tips into your routine, you can establish a sustainable and health-conscious approach to post-gastric sleeve surgery nutrition. Regularly reassessing and adjusting your meal plans based on your evolving needs ensures continued success on your health and wellness journey.

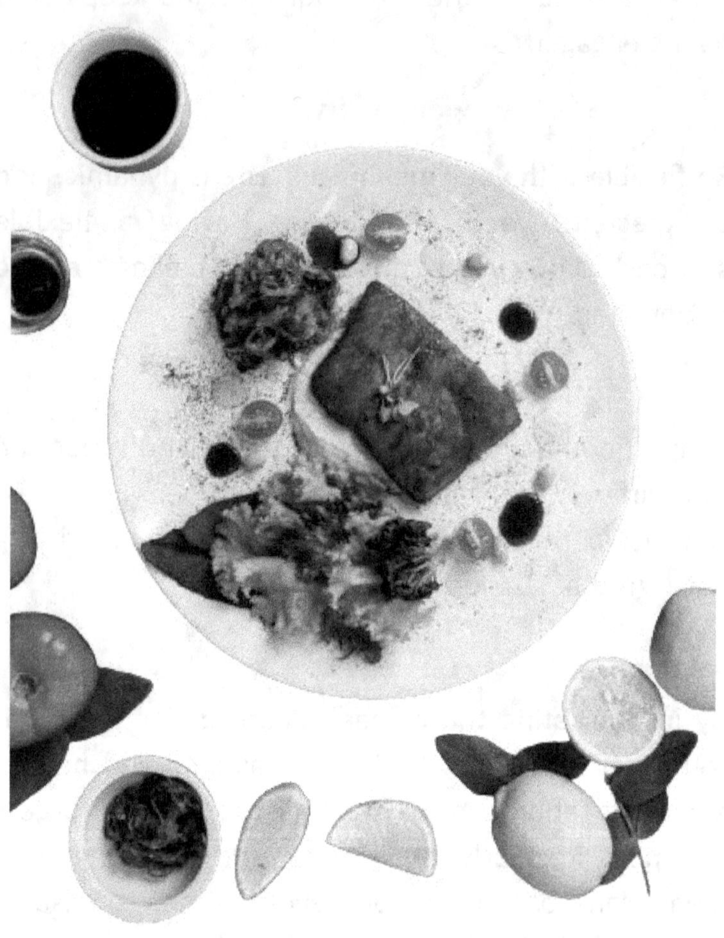

CHAPTER 3

Breakfasts for a Healthy Start

Protein-Packed Smoothies:

1. Berry Blast Protein Smoothie

Ingredients:

- 1/2 cup mixed berries (strawberries, blueberries, raspberries)
- 1/2 cup unsweetened almond milk
- 1/2 cup Greek yogurt (low-fat)
- 1 scoop vanilla protein powder
- Ice cubes (optional)

Preparation:

1. Blend berries, almond milk, Greek yogurt, and protein powder until smooth.
2. Add ice cubes if desired and blend again until well combined.
3. Pour into a glass and enjoy!

Servings: 1

Nutritional Value (approx.):

- Calories: 200

- Protein: 25g

- Carbohydrates: 15g

- Fat: 5g

- Fiber: 5g

Cooking Time: 5 minutes

2. Green Goddess Protein Smoothie

Ingredients:

- 1/2 cup spinach leaves

- 1/2 cucumber, peeled and sliced

- 1/2 avocado

- 1/2 cup unsweetened coconut water

- 1 scoop plant-based protein powder

- Mint leaves for garnish

Preparation:

1. Blend spinach, cucumber, avocado, coconut water, and protein powder until smooth.

2. Pour into a glass, garnish with mint leaves, and serve.

Servings: 1

Nutritional Value (approx.):

- Calories: 220

- Protein: 20g

- Carbohydrates: 12g

- Fat: 10g

- Fiber: 8g

Cooking Time: 5 minutes

3. Tropical Paradise Protein Smoothie

Ingredients:

- 1/2 cup pineapple chunks

- 1/2 banana

- 1/2 cup coconut milk (unsweetened)

- 1 scoop vanilla protein powder

- Ice cubes (optional)

Preparation:

1. Blend pineapple, banana, coconut milk, and protein powder until smooth.

2. Add ice cubes if desired and blend again until well combined.

3. Pour into a glass and transport yourself to a tropical paradise!

Servings: 1

Nutritional Value (approx.):

- Calories: 220

- Protein: 22g

- Carbohydrates: 20g

- Fat: 7g

- Fiber: 3g

Cooking Time: 5 minutes

4. Chocolate Peanut Butter Power Smoothie

Ingredients:

- 1 cup unsweetened almond milk
- 1 tablespoon natural peanut butter
- 1 tablespoon cocoa powder
- 1 scoop chocolate protein powder
- Ice cubes (optional)

Preparation:

1. Blend almond milk, peanut butter, cocoa powder, and chocolate protein powder until smooth.
2. Add ice cubes if desired and blend again until well combined.
3. Pour into a glass and indulge in this chocolatey treat.

Servings: 1

Nutritional Value (approx.): Calories: 250, Protein: 28g

- Carbohydrates: 10g
- Fat: 12g
- Fiber: 5g

Cooking Time: 5 minutes

5. Vanilla Almond Delight Smoothie

Ingredients:

- 1/2 cup unsweetened almond milk
- 1/2 cup cottage cheese (low-fat)
- 1/2 teaspoon almond extract
- 1 scoop vanilla protein powder
- 1/4 cup sliced almonds

Preparation:

1. Blend almond milk, cottage cheese, almond extract, and vanilla protein powder until smooth.

2. Top with sliced almonds for added crunch and nutrition.

3. Pour into a glass and savor the delightful combination of vanilla and almond.

Servings: 1

Nutritional Value (approx.): Calories: 230, Protein: 26g

- Carbohydrates: 8g
- Fat: 10g
- Fiber: 2g

Cooking Time: 5 minutes

Ingredients:

- 1/2 cup canned pumpkin (unsweetened)
- 1/2 teaspoon pumpkin spice
- 1/2 cup unsweetened almond milk
- 1 scoop vanilla protein powder
- Ice cubes (optional)

Preparation:

1. Blend pumpkin, pumpkin spice, almond milk, and vanilla protein powder until smooth.
2. Add ice cubes if desired and blend again until well combined.
3. Pour into a glass and enjoy the cozy flavors of pumpkin spice.

Servings: 1

Nutritional Value (approx.): Calories: 180, Protein: 20g, Carbohydrates: 15g, Fat: 5g, Fiber: 5g

Cooking Time: 5 minutes

These protein-packed smoothie recipes are not only delicious but also designed to align with bariatric-friendly, heart-healthy, kidney-friendly, and diabetes-friendly dietary considerations.

Energizing Oatmeal Variations

1. Apple Cinnamon Protein Oats:

Ingredients:

- 1/2 cup rolled oats
- 1/2 cup unsweetened almond milk
- 1/2 medium apple, diced
- 1 scoop vanilla protein powder
- 1/2 teaspoon cinnamon
- 1 tablespoon chopped walnuts (optional)

Instructions:

1. In a saucepan, combine oats, almond milk, and diced apples.
2. Cook over medium heat, stirring occasionally, until oats are cooked and apples are tender.
3. Stir in protein powder and cinnamon.
4. Top with chopped walnuts if desired.
5. Serve warm.

Servings: 1 | Nutritional Value (approx.): Calories: 350, Protein: 25g, Carbohydrates: 40g, Fat: 10g

Cooking Time: 10 minutes

2. Berries and Cream Oatmeal Bowl:

Ingredients:

- 1/2 cup old-fashioned oats

- 1/2 cup unsweetened almond milk

- 1/2 cup mixed berries (strawberries, blueberries, raspberries)

- 1 tablespoon Greek yogurt

- 1 teaspoon chia seeds

- 1/2 teaspoon vanilla extract

Instructions:

1. Cook oats with almond milk until desired consistency is reached.

2. Mix in vanilla extract.

3. Top with mixed berries, Greek yogurt, and chia seeds.

4. Drizzle with a touch of honey if desired.

5. Enjoy warm.

Servings: 1 | Nutritional Value (approx.): Calories: 300, Protein: 15g, Carbohydrates: 45g, Fat: 8g

Cooking Time: 8 minutes

Ingredients:

- 1/2 cup quick oats
- 1/2 cup unsweetened almond milk
- 2 tablespoons pumpkin puree
- 1 scoop vanilla protein powder
- 1/2 teaspoon pumpkin spice
- 1 tablespoon chopped pecans (optional)

Instructions:

1. Cook oats and almond milk until creamy.
2. Stir in pumpkin puree, protein powder, and pumpkin spice.
3. Top with chopped pecans if desired.
4. Serve warm.

Servings: 1 | Nutritional Value (approx.):

- Calories: 320
- Protein: 25g
- Carbohydrates: 35g
- Fat: 10g

Cooking Time: 7 minutes

Ingredients:

- 1/2 cup steel-cut oats
- 1/2 cup coconut milk (unsweetened)
- 1 tablespoon unsweetened cocoa powder
- 1 tablespoon almond butter
- 1 tablespoon shredded coconut (unsweetened)
- 1/2 teaspoon almond extract

Instructions:

1. Cook steel-cut oats with coconut milk until tender.
2. Stir in cocoa powder, almond butter, and almond extract.
3. Top with shredded coconut and enjoy warm.

Servings: 1 | Nutritional Value (approx.):

- Calories: 380
- Protein: 12g
- Carbohydrates: 40g
- Fat: 20g

Cooking Time: 15 minutes

5. Banana Nut Protein Oatmeal:

Ingredients:

- 1/2 cup rolled oats
- 1/2 cup almond milk
- 1/2 ripe banana, mashed
- 1 scoop vanilla protein powder
- 1 tablespoon chopped almonds
- 1/2 teaspoon cinnamon

Instructions:

1. Cook oats with almond milk until creamy.
2. Stir in mashed banana, protein powder, and cinnamon.
3. Top with chopped almonds.
4. Serve warm.

Servings: 1 | Nutritional Value (approx.):

- Calories: 330
- Protein: 22g
- Carbohydrates: 40g
- Fat: 10g

Cooking Time: 8 minutes

6. Chia Seed and Raspberry Overnight Oats:

Ingredients:

- 1/2 cup old-fashioned oats
- 1/2 cup unsweetened almond milk
- 1/2 cup fresh raspberries
- 1 tablespoon chia seeds
- 1 tablespoon slivered almonds
- 1/2 teaspoon vanilla extract

Instructions:

1. Mix oats, almond milk, raspberries, chia seeds, and vanilla extract in a jar.
2. Refrigerate overnight.
3. In the morning, top with slivered almonds and additional raspberries if desired.
4. Enjoy chilled.

Servings: 1 | Nutritional Value (approx.): Calories: 290, Protein: 10g, Carbohydrates: 35g, Fat: 12g

Prep Time: 5 minutes | Refrigeration Time: Overnight

These delicious and bariatric-friendly oatmeal variations provide a mix of flavors and nutrients to start your day on a healthy and satisfying note.

Egg-based Delights:

1. Spinach and Feta Egg Muffins:

Ingredients:

- 6 large eggs
- 1 cup fresh spinach, chopped
- 1/2 cup feta cheese, crumbled
- 1/4 cup cherry tomatoes, diced
- Salt and pepper to taste

Instructions:

1. Preheat the oven to 350°F (175°C).
2. In a bowl, whisk the eggs and season with salt and pepper.
3. Add chopped spinach, feta cheese, and diced cherry tomatoes to the egg mixture. Mix well.
4. Grease a muffin tin and pour the mixture evenly into each cup.
5. Bake for 15-20 minutes or until the eggs are set.
6. Allow the muffins to cool slightly before serving.

Servings: 3

Nutritional Value (per serving):

- Calories: 180
- Protein: 15g
- Carbohydrates: 3g
- Fat: 12g
- Fiber: 1g
- Sugar: 1g

Cooking Time: 20 minutes

2. Veggie-Packed Scrambled Eggs:

Ingredients:

- 4 large eggs
- 1/2 cup bell peppers, diced
- 1/2 cup zucchini, diced
- 1/4 cup red onion, finely chopped
- 1 tablespoon olive oil
- Salt and pepper to taste

Instructions:

1. Heat olive oil in a pan over medium heat.

2. Add diced bell peppers, zucchini, and red onion. Sauté until vegetables are tender.

3. In a bowl, whisk the eggs and season with salt and pepper.

4. Pour the eggs into the pan with the vegetables, stirring continuously until eggs are cooked.

5. Serve hot.

Servings: 2

Nutritional Value (per serving):

- Calories: 220

- Protein: 12g

- Carbohydrates: 8g

- Fat: 16g

- Fiber: 2g

- Sugar: 4g

Cooking Time: 15 minutes

3. Mushroom and Spinach Omelette:

Ingredients:

- 3 large eggs
- 1/2 cup mushrooms, sliced
- 1 cup fresh spinach
- 1/4 cup Swiss cheese, shredded
- Salt and pepper to taste

Instructions:

1. In a bowl, whisk the eggs and season with salt and pepper.
2. Sauté sliced mushrooms in a non-stick pan until they release moisture.
3. Add fresh spinach to the pan and cook until wilted.
4. Pour the whisked eggs over the mushrooms and spinach.
5. Sprinkle shredded Swiss cheese over the eggs and cook until the omelette is set.
6. Fold the omelette in half and serve.

Servings: 1

Nutritional Value:

- Calories: 250

- Protein: 20g

- Carbohydrates: 5g

- Fat: 18g

- Fiber: 2g

- Sugar: 1g

Cooking Time: 10 minutes

4. Caprese Breakfast Skillet:

Ingredients:

- 4 large eggs

- 1 cup cherry tomatoes, halved

- 1/2 cup fresh mozzarella, diced

- Fresh basil leaves

- 1 tablespoon olive oil

- Salt and pepper to taste

Instructions:

1. Heat olive oil in a skillet over medium heat.

2. Add cherry tomatoes and cook until softened.

3. Crack the eggs over the tomatoes, allowing them to cook to your preferred doneness.

4. Sprinkle diced mozzarella over the eggs.

5. Season with salt and pepper and garnish with fresh basil leaves.

6. Serve immediately.

Servings: 2

Nutritional Value (per serving):

- Calories: 280

- Protein: 16g

- Carbohydrates: 5g

- Fat: 21g

- Fiber: 1g

- Sugar: 2g

Cooking Time: 15 minutes

Ingredients:

- 6 large eggs
- 1/2 cup smoked salmon, chopped
- 1/4 cup cream cheese, softened
- 1/4 cup chives, chopped
- Salt and pepper to taste

Instructions:

1. Preheat the oven to 375°F (190°C).
2. In a bowl, whisk the eggs and season with salt and pepper.
3. Add chopped smoked salmon, softened cream cheese, and chopped chives to the eggs. Mix well.
4. Grease a baking dish and pour the egg mixture into it.
5. Bake for 20-25 minutes or until the frittata is set.
6. Allow it to cool slightly before slicing and serving.

Servings: 4

Nutritional Value (per serving):

- Calories: 220

- Protein: 18g

- Carbohydrates: 2g

- Fat: 15g

- Fiber: 0g

- Sugar: 1g

Cooking Time: 25 minutes

6. Mediterranean Egg Muffins:

Ingredients:

- 6 large eggs

- 1/2 cup black olives, sliced

- 1/4 cup feta cheese, crumbled

- 1/4 cup sun-dried tomatoes, chopped

- 1/4 cup fresh basil, chopped

- Salt and pepper to taste

Instructions:

1. Preheat the oven to 350°F (175°C).

2. In a bowl, whisk the eggs and season with salt and pepper.

3. Add sliced black olives, crumbled feta cheese, chopped sun-dried tomatoes, and chopped fresh basil to the eggs. Mix well.

4. Grease a muffin tin and pour the mixture evenly into each cup.

5. Bake for 15-20 minutes or until the eggs are set.

6. Allow the muffins to cool slightly before serving.

Servings: 3

Nutritional Value (per serving):

- Calories: 200

- Protein: 12g

- Carbohydrates: 5g

- Fat: 15g

- Fiber: 1g

- Sugar: 2g

Cooking Time: 20 minutes

CHAPTER 4

Wholesome Lunches and Satisfying Soups

Lean Protein Salads:

1. Grilled Chicken and Avocado Salad:

Ingredients:

- 2 boneless, skinless chicken breasts
- 4 cups mixed salad greens
- 1 avocado, sliced
- 1 cup cherry tomatoes, halved
- 1/4 cup red onion, thinly sliced
- 2 tablespoons olive oil
- 1 tablespoon balsamic vinegar
- Salt and pepper to taste

Instructions:

1. Season chicken breasts with salt and pepper.
2. Grill the chicken until fully cooked, then slice.

3. In a large bowl, combine salad greens, sliced avocado, cherry tomatoes, and red onion.

4. Top the salad with grilled chicken slices.

5. In a small bowl, whisk together olive oil and balsamic vinegar. Drizzle over the salad.

6. Toss gently and serve.

Servings: 2

Nutritional Value (per serving):

- Calories: 350

- Protein: 25g

- Carbohydrates: 12g

- Fat: 22g

- Fiber: 7g

- Sugar: 3g

Cooking Time: 15 minutes

Ingredients:

- 1 can (5 oz) tuna, drained
- 1 can (15 oz) white beans, drained and rinsed
- 2 cups arugula
- 1/2 cup cucumber, sliced
- 1/4 cup red bell pepper, diced
- 2 tablespoons lemon juice
- 1 tablespoon olive oil
- 1 teaspoon Dijon mustard
- Salt and pepper to taste

Instructions:

1. In a large bowl, combine tuna, white beans, arugula, cucumber, and red bell pepper.

2. In a small bowl, whisk together lemon juice, olive oil, Dijon mustard, salt, and pepper.

3. Pour the dressing over the salad and toss gently to combine.

4. Serve immediately.

Servings: 3

Nutritional Value (per serving):

- Calories: 280

- Protein: 20g

- Carbohydrates: 30g

- Fat: 10g

- Fiber: 9g

- Sugar: 2g

Cooking Time: 10 minutes

---

3. Shrimp and Quinoa Salad:

Ingredients:

- 1 cup cooked quinoa

- 8 oz shrimp, peeled and deveined

- 2 cups mixed salad greens

- 1 cup cherry tomatoes, halved

- 1/2 cup cucumber, diced

- 1/4 cup feta cheese, crumbled

- 2 tablespoons olive oil

- 1 tablespoon lemon juice

- 1 clove garlic, minced

- Salt and pepper to taste

Instructions:

1. Season shrimp with salt and pepper.

2. In a pan, sauté shrimp until fully cooked.

3. In a large bowl, combine cooked quinoa, salad greens, cherry tomatoes, cucumber, and feta cheese.

4. Top the salad with cooked shrimp.

5. In a small bowl, whisk together olive oil, lemon juice, minced garlic, salt, and pepper.

6. Drizzle the dressing over the salad and toss gently.

Servings: 2

Nutritional Value (per serving): Calories: 320, Protein: 25g, Carbohydrates: 25g, Fat: 15g, Fiber: 4g, Sugar: 3g

Cooking Time: 20 minutes

4. Turkey and Quinoa Stuffed Bell Peppers:

Ingredients:

- 2 bell peppers, halved and seeds removed
- 1 cup cooked quinoa
- 8 oz ground turkey
- 1/2 cup black beans, drained and rinsed
- 1/2 cup corn kernels
- 1/4 cup salsa
- 1 teaspoon chili powder
- 1/2 teaspoon cumin
- Salt and pepper to taste
- 1/4 cup shredded cheddar cheese (optional, for topping)

Instructions:

1. Preheat the oven to 375°F (190°C).

2. In a pan, cook ground turkey until browned. Season with chili powder, cumin, salt, and pepper.

3. In a bowl, mix cooked quinoa, black beans, corn, salsa, and cooked turkey.

4. Stuff the bell peppers with the quinoa and turkey mixture.

5. If desired, top each stuffed pepper with shredded cheddar cheese.

6. Bake for 25-30 minutes or until peppers are tender.

Servings: 2

Nutritional Value (per serving):

- Calories: 350

- Protein: 25g

- Carbohydrates: 30g

- Fat: 15g

- Fiber: 6g

- Sugar: 3g

Cooking Time: 30 minutes

Ingredients:

- 2 salmon fillets
- 1 bunch asparagus, trimmed
- 4 cups mixed salad greens
- 1/4 cup cherry tomatoes, halved
- 1/4 cup red onion, thinly sliced
- 2 tablespoons olive oil
- 1 tablespoon balsamic vinegar
- Salt and pepper to taste
- Lemon wedges for serving

Instructions:

1. Preheat the oven to 400°F (200°C).
2. Place salmon fillets and trimmed asparagus on a baking sheet.
3. Drizzle olive oil over salmon and asparagus. Season with salt and pepper.
4. Roast in the oven for 15-20 minutes or until salmon is cooked through.

5. In a large bowl, combine salad greens, cherry tomatoes, and sliced red onion.

6. Top the salad with roasted salmon and asparagus.

7. Drizzle balsamic vinegar over the salad and serve with lemon wedges.

Servings: 2

Nutritional Value (per serving):

- Calories: 320

- Protein: 25g

- Carbohydrates: 15g

- Fat: 18g

- Fiber: 6g

- Sugar: 4g

Cooking Time: 20 minutes

Ingredients:

- 2 boneless, skinless chicken breasts
- 4 cups romaine lettuce, chopped
- 1 cucumber, diced
- 1 cup cherry tomatoes, halved
- 1/4 cup Kalamata olives, sliced
- 1/4 cup feta cheese, crumbled
- 2 tablespoons olive oil
- 1 tablespoon red wine vinegar
- 1 teaspoon dried oregano
- Salt and pepper to taste

Instructions:

1. Season chicken breasts with dried oregano, salt, and pepper.

2. Grill or cook chicken until fully cooked, then slice.

3. In a large bowl, combine chopped romaine lettuce, diced cucumber, cherry tomatoes,

sliced Kalamata olives, and crumbled feta cheese.

4. Top the salad with sliced grilled chicken.

5. In a small bowl, whisk together olive oil and red wine vinegar. Drizzle over the salad.

6. Toss gently and serve.

Servings: 2

Nutritional Value (per serving):

- Calories: 280

- Protein: 25g

- Carbohydrates: 10g

- Fat: 16g

- Fiber: 4g

- Sugar: 4g

Cooking Time: 15 minutes

These lean protein salads are not only bariatric-friendly but also suitable for individuals managing diabetes, heart disease, kidney health, and weight loss. Adjust portion sizes based on your dietary.

Nourishing Soups for Recovery:

1. Chicken and Vegetable Broth:

Ingredients:

- 2 boneless, skinless chicken breasts
- 6 cups low-sodium chicken broth
- 2 carrots, sliced
- 2 celery stalks, chopped
- 1 cup green beans, chopped
- 1/2 cup quinoa, rinsed
- 1 teaspoon dried thyme
- Salt and pepper to taste
- Fresh parsley for garnish

Instructions:

1. In a large pot, bring chicken broth to a simmer.
2. Add chicken breasts, carrots, celery, green beans, quinoa, dried thyme, salt, and pepper.
3. Simmer for 20-25 minutes or until chicken is cooked through.

4. Remove chicken, shred it, and return it to the pot.

5. Garnish with fresh parsley before serving.

Servings: 4

Nutritional Value (per serving):

- Calories: 220

- Protein: 25g

- Carbohydrates: 18g

- Fat: 5g

- Fiber: 3g

- Sugar: 2g

Cooking Time: 25 minutes

2. Lentil and Spinach Soup:

Ingredients:

- 1 cup dried green lentils, rinsed

- 1 onion, diced

- 2 carrots, diced

- 2 celery stalks, diced

- 3 cloves garlic, minced

- 6 cups vegetable broth

- 2 cups fresh spinach

- 1 teaspoon cumin

- 1 teaspoon paprika

- Salt and pepper to taste

- Lemon wedges for serving

Instructions:

1. In a large pot, sauté onion, carrots, celery, and garlic until softened.

2. Add lentils, vegetable broth, cumin, paprika, salt, and pepper.

3. Simmer for 25-30 minutes or until lentils are tender.

4. Stir in fresh spinach and cook until wilted.

5. Serve with a squeeze of lemon.

Servings: 6

Nutritional Value (per serving):

- Calories: 180

- Protein: 12g

- Carbohydrates: 30g

- Fat: 1g

- Fiber: 9g

- Sugar: 3g

Cooking Time: 30 minutes

---

3. Turkey and Vegetable Soup:

Ingredients:

- 1 lb ground turkey

- 1 onion, chopped

- 2 carrots, sliced

- 2 zucchini, diced

- 3 cloves garlic, minced

- 6 cups low-sodium chicken broth

- 1 can (14 oz) diced tomatoes

- 1 teaspoon Italian seasoning

- Salt and pepper to taste

- Fresh basil for garnish

Instructions:

1. In a large pot, brown ground turkey and onions until turkey is cooked.

2. Add carrots, zucchini, garlic, chicken broth, diced tomatoes, Italian seasoning, salt, and pepper.

3. Simmer for 20-25 minutes.

4. Garnish with fresh basil before serving.

Servings: 5

Nutritional Value (per serving):

- Calories: 230

- Protein: 20g

- Carbohydrates: 15g

- Fat: 10g

- Fiber: 4g

- Sugar: 5g

Cooking Time: 25 minutes

Ingredients:

- 1 head cauliflower, chopped
- 2 leeks, sliced
- 3 cups vegetable broth
- 1 cup unsweetened almond milk
- 2 tablespoons olive oil
- 1 teaspoon thyme
- Salt and pepper to taste
- Chopped chives for garnish

Instructions:

1. In a pot, sauté leeks in olive oil until softened.
2. Add chopped cauliflower, vegetable broth, almond milk, thyme, salt, and pepper.
3. Simmer for 15-20 minutes or until cauliflower is tender.
4. Blend the soup until smooth using an immersion blender.
5. Garnish with chopped chives before serving.

Servings: 4

Nutritional Value (per serving):

- Calories: 150

- Protein: 4g

- Carbohydrates: 14g

- Fat: 10g

- Fiber: 5g

- Sugar: 4g

Cooking Time: 20 minutes

---

5. Spinach and Chickpea Stew:

Ingredients:

- 1 can (15 oz) chickpeas, drained and rinsed

- 1 onion, chopped

- 3 cloves garlic, minced

- 4 cups vegetable broth

- 4 cups fresh spinach

- 1 can (14 oz) diced tomatoes

- 1 teaspoon cumin

- 1 teaspoon smoked paprika

- Salt and pepper to taste

- Lemon wedges for serving

Instructions:

1. In a pot, sauté onion and garlic until softened.

2. Add chickpeas, vegetable broth, spinach, diced tomatoes, cumin, smoked paprika, salt, and pepper.

3. Simmer for 15-20 minutes.

4. Serve with a squeeze of lemon.

Servings: 4

Nutritional Value (per serving):

- Calories: 200

- Protein: 10g

- Carbohydrates: 30g

- Fat: 5g

- Fiber: 8g

- Sugar: 5g

Cooking Time: 20 minutes

Ingredients:

- 6 ripe tomatoes, chopped
- 1 onion, chopped
- 3 cloves garlic, minced
- 4 cups low-sodium vegetable broth
- 1/4 cup fresh basil, chopped
- 2 tablespoons olive oil
- Salt and pepper to taste
- Greek yogurt for garnish

Instructions:

1. In a pot, sauté onion and garlic in olive oil until softened.
2. Add chopped tomatoes, vegetable broth, fresh basil, salt, and pepper.
3. Simmer for 25-30 minutes.
4. Blend the soup until smooth using an immersion blender.
5. Serve with a dollop of Greek yogurt.

Servings: 4

Nutritional Value (per serving):

- Calories: 180

- Protein: 5g

- Carbohydrates: 20g

- Fat: 10g

- Fiber: 5g

- Sugar: 8g

Cooking Time: 30 minutes

These nourishing soup recipes are designed to be bariatric-friendly and suitable for individuals managing diabetes, heart disease, kidney health, and weight loss.

Creative Lunch Wraps:

1. Turkey and Veggie Collard Wraps:

Ingredients:

- 4 large collard green leaves
- 1/2 lb turkey breast slices
- 1/2 cup hummus
- 1 cucumber, julienned
- 1 carrot, julienned
- 1/4 cup alfalfa sprouts
- Salt and pepper to taste

Instructions:

1. Blanch collard green leaves in boiling water for 30 seconds. Pat them dry.

2. Lay each collard leaf flat and spread hummus on it.

3. Place turkey slices, cucumber, carrot, and alfalfa sprouts along the center of each leaf.

4. Season with salt and pepper.

5. Fold in the sides and roll up the wraps tightly.

6. Secure with toothpicks if needed and slice in half before serving.

Servings: 2

Nutritional Value (per serving):

- Calories: 250

- Protein: 25g

- Carbohydrates: 20g

- Fat: 8g

- Fiber: 8g

- Sugar: 4g

Preparation Time: 15 minutes

---

2. Grilled Chicken Caesar Lettuce Wraps:

Ingredients:

- 4 large Romaine lettuce leaves

- 1/2 lb grilled chicken breast, sliced

- 1/4 cup Caesar dressing (low-fat)

- 1/4 cup cherry tomatoes, halved

- 2 tablespoons grated Parmesan cheese

- Freshly ground black pepper to taste

Instructions:

1. Lay Romaine lettuce leaves flat.

2. Place grilled chicken slices on each leaf.

3. Drizzle Caesar dressing over the chicken.

4. Add cherry tomatoes and sprinkle Parmesan cheese.

5. Finish with freshly ground black pepper.

6. Roll up the wraps and secure with toothpicks if desired.

Servings: 2

Nutritional Value (per serving):

- Calories: 280

- Protein: 30g

- Carbohydrates: 8g

- Fat: 12g

- Fiber: 3g

- Sugar: 2g

Preparation Time: 20 minutes

Ingredients:

- 2 large whole wheat tortillas
- 1 avocado, sliced
- 1 cup black beans, drained and rinsed
- 1/2 cup corn kernels
- 1/4 cup red onion, finely chopped
- 2 tablespoons lime juice
- Fresh cilantro for garnish
- Salt and pepper to taste

Instructions:

1. Lay out tortillas and divide avocado slices between them.

2. In a bowl, mix black beans, corn, and red onion. Season with lime juice, salt, and pepper.

3. Spoon the black bean mixture over the avocado.

4. Garnish with fresh cilantro.

5. Roll up the wraps tightly and slice before serving.

Servings: 2

Nutritional Value (per serving):

- Calories: 320
- Protein: 10g
- Carbohydrates: 40g
- Fat: 15g
- Fiber: 10g
- Sugar: 2g

Preparation Time: 15 minutes

---

4. Smoked Salmon and Greek Yogurt Wrap:

Ingredients:

- 2 whole wheat wraps
- 4 oz smoked salmon
- 1/2 cup Greek yogurt
- 1 cucumber, thinly sliced
- 1 tablespoon capers
- Fresh dill for garnish
- Lemon wedges for serving

Instructions:

1. Lay out the wraps and spread Greek yogurt
    evenly on each.

2. Place smoked salmon on top of the yogurt.

3. Add cucumber slices and sprinkle capers.

4. Garnish with fresh dill.

5. Roll up the wraps tightly and serve with lemon
    wedges.

Servings: 2

Nutritional Value (per serving):

- Calories: 280

- Protein: 25g

- Carbohydrates: 20g

- Fat: 12g

- Fiber: 3g

- Sugar: 4g

Preparation Time: 10 minutes

5. Veggie and Hummus Wrap:

Ingredients:

- 2 spinach tortillas
- 1/2 cup hummus
- 1 cup mixed bell peppers, thinly sliced
- 1/2 cup cherry tomatoes, halved
- 1/4 cup red onion, thinly sliced
- 1/4 cup feta cheese, crumbled
- Fresh basil leaves for garnish

Instructions:

1. Spread hummus evenly on each tortilla.
2. Layer bell peppers, cherry tomatoes, red onion, and feta cheese.
3. Garnish with fresh basil leaves.
4. Roll up the wraps tightly and slice before serving.

Servings: 2

Nutritional Value (per serving):

- Calories: 240

- Protein: 8g

- Carbohydrates: 30g

- Fat: 10g

- Fiber: 5g

- Sugar: 4g

Preparation Time: 15 minutes

6. Quinoa and Veggie Wrap:

Ingredients:

- 2 whole wheat wraps

- 1 cup cooked quinoa

- 1/2 cup hummus

- 1/2 cup cucumber, diced

- 1/2 cup cherry tomatoes, quartered

- 1/4 cup red bell pepper, diced

- 1/4 cup black olives, sliced

- Fresh parsley for garnish

Instructions:

1. In a bowl, mix cooked quinoa, cucumber, cherry tomatoes, red bell pepper, and black olives.

2. Spread hummus evenly on each wrap.

3. Spoon the quinoa mixture onto the wraps.

4. Garnish with fresh parsley.

5. Roll up the wraps tightly and slice before serving.

Servings: 2

Nutritional Value (per serving):

- Calories: 280

- Protein: 10g

- Carbohydrates: 35g

- Fat: 10g

- Fiber: 6g

- Sugar: 3g

Preparation Time: 20 minutes

Chapter 5:

Flavorful Dinners for Stomach Health

Grilled Protein Specialties:

1. Lemon Herb Grilled Chicken:

Ingredients:

- 2 boneless, skinless chicken breasts
- 2 tablespoons olive oil
- 2 tablespoons lemon juice
- 1 teaspoon dried thyme
- 1 teaspoon dried rosemary
- Salt and pepper to taste

Instructions:

1. In a bowl, mix olive oil, lemon juice, thyme, rosemary, salt, and pepper.

2. Marinate chicken breasts in the mixture for at least 30 minutes.

3. Preheat grill to medium-high heat.

4. Grill chicken for 6-8 minutes per side or until fully cooked.

5. Serve with a side of steamed vegetables.

Servings: 2

Nutritional Value (per serving):

- Calories: 250

- Protein: 30g

- Carbohydrates: 2g

- Fat: 14g

- Fiber: 1g

- Sugar: 0g

Cooking Time: 20 minutes

---

2. Garlic and Herb Grilled Salmon:

Ingredients:

- 2 salmon fillets

- 2 tablespoons olive oil

- 3 cloves garlic, minced

- 1 teaspoon dried thyme

- 1 teaspoon dried oregano

- Salt and pepper to taste

- Lemon wedges for serving

Instructions:

1. Mix olive oil, minced garlic, thyme, oregano, salt, and pepper in a bowl.

2. Rub the mixture over salmon fillets and let them marinate for 15-20 minutes.

3. Preheat grill to medium heat.

4. Grill salmon for 4-5 minutes per side or until flakes easily with a fork.

5. Serve with lemon wedges and a side of roasted vegetables.

Servings: 2

Nutritional Value (per serving):

- Calories: 300

- Protein: 25g

- Carbohydrates: 1g

- Fat: 20g

- Fiber: 0g

- Sugar: 0g

Cooking Time: 15 minutes

3. Cilantro Lime Grilled Shrimp:

Ingredients:

- 1 lb large shrimp, peeled and deveined
- 2 tablespoons olive oil
- 2 tablespoons fresh cilantro, chopped
- 1 tablespoon lime juice
- 1 teaspoon cumin
- Salt and pepper to taste

Instructions:

1. In a bowl, combine olive oil, chopped cilantro, lime juice, cumin, salt, and pepper.
2. Toss shrimp in the marinade and let them sit for 15-20 minutes.
3. Preheat grill to medium-high heat.
4. Grill shrimp for 2-3 minutes per side or until opaque.
5. Serve with a side of quinoa or cauliflower rice.

Servings: 4

Nutritional Value (per serving):

- Calories: 150

- Protein: 20g

- Carbohydrates: 1g

- Fat: 7g

- Fiber: 0g

- Sugar: 0g

Cooking Time: 10 minutes

4. Herb-Marinated Turkey Burgers:

Ingredients:

- 1 lb ground turkey

- 2 tablespoons fresh parsley, chopped

- 1 tablespoon fresh thyme, chopped

- 1 tablespoon Dijon mustard

- 1 clove garlic, minced

- Salt and pepper to taste

- Whole wheat burger buns

- Lettuce, tomato, and red onion for toppings

Instructions:

1. In a bowl, mix ground turkey, chopped parsley, thyme, Dijon mustard, minced garlic, salt, and pepper.

2. Form the mixture into burger patties.

3. Preheat grill to medium heat.

4. Grill turkey burgers for 5-6 minutes per side or until fully cooked.

5. Serve on whole wheat buns with desired toppings.

Servings: 4

Nutritional Value (per serving):

- Calories: 250

- Protein: 30g

- Carbohydrates: 20g

- Fat: 10g

- Fiber: 3g

- Sugar: 1g

Cooking Time: 15 minutes

Ingredients:

- 1 block extra-firm tofu, pressed and cubed
- 1/4 cup low-sodium soy sauce
- 2 tablespoons honey or maple syrup
- 1 tablespoon rice vinegar
- 1 teaspoon sesame oil
- 2 cloves garlic, minced
- 1 teaspoon grated ginger
- Wooden skewers, soaked in water
- Sesame seeds and green onions for garnish

Instructions:

1. In a bowl, whisk together soy sauce, honey or maple syrup, rice vinegar, sesame oil, minced garlic, and grated ginger.

2. Thread tofu cubes onto soaked wooden skewers.

3. Brush the teriyaki sauce over the tofu skewers.

4. Preheat grill to medium-high heat.

5. Grill tofu skewers for 3-4 minutes per side or until grill marks appear.

6. Garnish with sesame seeds and chopped green onions before serving.

Servings: 3

Nutritional Value (per serving):

- Calories: 180

- Protein: 12g

- Carbohydrates: 15g

- Fat: 8g

- Fiber: 2g

- Sugar: 8g

Cooking Time: 15 minutes

Ingredients:

- Assorted vegetables (bell peppers, cherry tomatoes, zucchini, mushrooms)

- 2 tablespoons balsamic vinegar

- 1 tablespoon olive oil

- 1 teaspoon dried basil

- 1 teaspoon dried oregano

- Salt and pepper to taste

Instructions:

1. In a bowl, whisk together balsamic vinegar, olive oil, dried basil, dried oregano, salt, and pepper.

2. Thread assorted vegetables onto skewers.

3. Brush the balsamic glaze over the vegetable skewers.

4. Preheat grill to medium heat.

5. Grill vegetable skewers for 10-12 minutes or until vegetables are tender.

6. Serve as a side dish or with a lean protein of your choice.

Servings: 4

Nutritional Value (per serving):

- Calories: 80
- Protein: 2g
- Carbohydrates: 12g
- Fat: 3g
- Fiber: 4g
- Sugar: 7g

Cooking Time: 15 minutes

1. Herb-Crusted Baked Chicken Breast:

Ingredients:

- 2 boneless, skinless chicken breasts

- 2 tablespoons olive oil

- 1 tablespoon fresh parsley, chopped

- 1 teaspoon dried thyme

- 1 teaspoon garlic powder

- Salt and pepper to taste

Instructions:

1. Preheat the oven to 400°F (200°C).

2. Mix olive oil, chopped parsley, thyme, garlic powder, salt, and pepper in a bowl.

3. Coat each chicken breast with the herb mixture.

4. Place the chicken breasts on a baking sheet.

5. Bake for 20-25 minutes or until the internal temperature reaches 165°F (74°C).

6. Serve with roasted vegetables or a side salad.

Servings: 2

Nutritional Value (per serving):

- Calories: 250

- Protein: 30g

- Carbohydrates: 1g

- Fat: 14g

- Fiber: 0g

- Sugar: 0g

Cooking Time: 25 minutes

---

2. Baked Lemon Garlic Salmon:

Ingredients:

- 2 salmon fillets

- 2 tablespoons olive oil

- 2 tablespoons lemon juice

- 2 cloves garlic, minced

- 1 teaspoon dried dill

- Salt and pepper to taste

Instructions:

1. Preheat the oven to 375°F (190°C).

2. Place salmon fillets on a baking dish.

3. Mix olive oil, lemon juice, minced garlic, dried dill, salt, and pepper in a bowl.

4. Pour the mixture over the salmon.

5. Bake for 15-20 minutes or until the salmon is cooked through.

6. Garnish with fresh lemon wedges and serve with steamed broccoli.

Servings: 2

Nutritional Value (per serving):

- Calories: 280

- Protein: 25g

- Carbohydrates: 2g

- Fat: 18g

- Fiber: 0g

- Sugar: 0g

Cooking Time: 20 minutes

3. Mediterranean Baked Cod:

Ingredients:

- 2 cod fillets

- 2 tablespoons olive oil

- 1 tablespoon lemon juice

- 1 teaspoon dried oregano

- 1/2 teaspoon paprika

- Salt and pepper to taste

- Cherry tomatoes, olives, and feta cheese for garnish

Instructions:

1. Preheat the oven to 375°F (190°C).

2. Place cod fillets in a baking dish.

3. Mix olive oil, lemon juice, dried oregano, paprika, salt, and pepper in a bowl.

4. Pour the mixture over the cod.

5. Bake for 15-20 minutes or until the fish flakes easily.

6. Garnish with cherry tomatoes, olives, and crumbled feta cheese before serving.

Servings: 2

Nutritional Value (per serving):

- Calories: 220

- Protein: 25g

- Carbohydrates: 4g

- Fat: 12g

- Fiber: 1g

- Sugar: 1g

Cooking Time: 20 minutes

---

4. Pesto Zoodle Bake:

Ingredients:

- 2 zucchinis, spiralized into zoodles

- 1 cup cherry tomatoes, halved

- 1/4 cup pesto sauce

- 1/4 cup grated Parmesan cheese

- Salt and pepper to taste

Instructions:

1. Preheat the oven to 375°F (190°C).

2. In a bowl, toss zoodles and cherry tomatoes with pesto sauce.

3. Transfer the mixture to a baking dish.

4. Sprinkle grated Parmesan cheese over the top.

5. Bake for 15-20 minutes or until zoodles are tender.

6. Season with salt and pepper before serving.

Servings: 2

Nutritional Value (per serving):

- Calories: 180

- Protein: 8g

- Carbohydrates: 8g

- Fat: 14g

- Fiber: 3g

- Sugar: 5g

Cooking Time: 20 minutes

Ingredients:

- 1 lb lean ground turkey
- 1/4 cup almond flour
- 1 egg
- 2 tablespoons fresh rosemary, chopped
- 1 teaspoon garlic powder
- Salt and pepper to taste
- Sugar-free marinara sauce for serving

Instructions:

1. Preheat the oven to 400°F (200°C).
2. In a bowl, combine ground turkey, almond flour, egg, chopped rosemary, garlic powder, salt, and pepper.
3. Form the mixture into meatballs and place them on a baking sheet.
4. Bake for 20-25 minutes or until the meatballs are cooked through.
5. Serve with sugar-free marinara sauce and steamed broccoli.

Servings: 4

Nutritional Value (per serving):

- Calories: 180

- Protein: 20g

- Carbohydrates: 2g

- Fat: 10g

- Fiber: 1g

- Sugar: 0g

Cooking Time: 25 minutes

---

6. Lemon Herb Baked Tofu:

Ingredients:

- 1 block extra-firm tofu, pressed and sliced

- 2 tablespoons olive oil

- 2 tablespoons lemon juice

- 1 tablespoon fresh parsley, chopped

- 1 teaspoon dried thyme

- Salt and pepper to taste

Instructions:

1. Preheat the oven to 375°F (190°C).

2. Mix olive oil, lemon juice, chopped parsley, dried thyme, salt, and pepper in a bowl.

3. Coat each tofu slice with the herb mixture.

4. Place the tofu slices on a baking sheet.

5. Bake for 20-25 minutes or until the tofu is golden brown.

6. Serve with a side of roasted Brussels sprouts.

Servings: 3

Nutritional Value (per serving):

- Calories: 150

- Protein: 10g

- Carbohydrates: 6g

- Fat: 10g

- Fiber: 2g

- Sugar: 1g

Cooking Time: 25 minutes

One-Pot Wonders:

1. Lemon Garlic Chicken Quinoa Bowl:

Ingredients:

- 1 lb boneless, skinless chicken thighs, cut into bite-sized pieces

- 1 cup quinoa, rinsed

- 2 cups low-sodium chicken broth

- 1 lemon, juiced and zested

- 3 cloves garlic, minced

- 1 teaspoon dried oregano

- Salt and pepper to taste

- Fresh parsley for garnish

Instructions:

1. In a large pot, brown chicken pieces over medium heat.

2. Add quinoa, chicken broth, lemon juice, lemon zest, minced garlic, dried oregano, salt, and pepper.

3. Bring to a boil, then reduce heat, cover, and simmer for 15-20 minutes or until quinoa is cooked and chicken is tender.

4. Garnish with fresh parsley before serving.

Servings: 4

Nutritional Value (per serving):

- Calories: 300

- Protein: 30g

- Carbohydrates: 30g

- Fat: 8g

- Fiber: 4g

- Sugar: 1g

Cooking Time: 30 minutes

---

2. Shrimp and Vegetable Stir-Fry Quinoa:

Ingredients:

- 1 lb shrimp, peeled and deveined

- 1 cup quinoa, rinsed

- 2 cups water

- 2 cups mixed vegetables (broccoli, bell peppers, snap peas)

- 2 tablespoons low-sodium soy sauce

- 1 tablespoon sesame oil

- 1 teaspoon fresh ginger, grated

- 2 cloves garlic, minced

- Green onions for garnish

Instructions:

1. In a pot, combine quinoa and water. Bring to a boil, then reduce heat, cover, and simmer for 15 minutes.

2. In a large skillet, sauté shrimp, mixed vegetables, soy sauce, sesame oil, grated ginger, and minced garlic until shrimp is cooked and vegetables are tender.

3. Mix in cooked quinoa and stir until well combined.

4. Garnish with green onions before serving.

Servings: 4

Nutritional Value (per serving): Calories: 280, Protein: 25g

- Carbohydrates: 30g

- Fat: 7g

- Fiber: 5g

- Sugar: 2g

Cooking Time: 25 minutes

Ingredients:

- 1 lb lean ground turkey
- 2 sweet potatoes, peeled and diced
- 1 can (15 oz) black beans, drained and rinsed
- 1 can (15 oz) diced tomatoes
- 1 onion, diced
- 2 cloves garlic, minced
- 2 tablespoons chili powder
- 1 teaspoon cumin
- Salt and pepper to taste
- Greek yogurt and cilantro for garnish

Instructions:

1. In a large pot, brown ground turkey over medium heat.

2. Add sweet potatoes, black beans, diced tomatoes, diced onion, minced garlic, chili powder, cumin, salt, and pepper.

3. Bring to a boil, then reduce heat and simmer for 20-25 minutes or until sweet potatoes are tender.

4. Serve with a dollop of Greek yogurt and garnish with cilantro.

Servings: 4

Nutritional Value (per serving):

- Calories: 320

- Protein: 30g

- Carbohydrates: 35g

- Fat: 8g

- Fiber: 8g

- Sugar: 8g

Cooking Time: 30 minutes

---

4. Lemon Herb Salmon and Asparagus Foil Packets:

Ingredients:

- 2 salmon fillets

- 1 bunch asparagus, trimmed

- 1 lemon, sliced

- 2 tablespoons olive oil

- 1 teaspoon dried dill

- Salt and pepper to taste

Instructions:

1. Preheat the oven to 400°F (200°C).

2. Place each salmon fillet on a piece of foil.

3. Arrange asparagus around the salmon and place lemon slices on top.

4. Drizzle olive oil over the salmon and asparagus. Sprinkle with dried dill, salt, and pepper.

5. Seal the foil packets and bake for 20-25 minutes or until salmon is cooked through.

6. Serve directly from the foil packets.

Servings: 2

Nutritional Value (per serving):

- Calories: 300

- Protein: 25g

- Carbohydrates: 10g

- Fat: 18g

- Fiber: 4g

- Sugar: 3g

Cooking Time: 25 minutes

Ingredients:

- 1 lb ground turkey

- 1 eggplant, diced

- 2 zucchinis, diced

- 1 bell pepper, diced

- 1 onion, diced

- 2 cloves garlic, minced

- 1 can (15 oz) diced tomatoes

- 2 tablespoons tomato paste

- 1 teaspoon dried thyme

- 1 teaspoon dried rosemary

- Salt and pepper to taste

- Fresh basil for garnish

Instructions:

1. In a large pot, brown ground turkey over medium heat.

2. Add diced eggplant, zucchinis, bell pepper, diced onion, minced garlic, diced tomatoes,

tomato paste, dried thyme, dried rosemary, salt, and pepper.

3. Simmer for 25-30 minutes or until vegetables are tender.

4. Garnish with fresh basil before serving.

Servings: 4

Nutritional Value (per serving):

- Calories: 280

- Protein: 25g

- Carbohydrates: 20g

- Fat: 12g

- Fiber: 6g

- Sugar: 8g

Cooking Time: 30 minutes

6. Chicken and Broccoli Alfredo Skillet:

Ingredients:

- 1 lb boneless, skinless chicken breasts, sliced

- 2 cups broccoli florets

- 2 cups cauliflower rice

- 1 cup unsweetened almond milk

- 1/2 cup grated Parmesan cheese

- 2 tablespoons nutritional yeast

- 1 teaspoon garlic powder

- Salt and pepper to taste

Instructions:

1. In a large skillet, cook sliced chicken over medium heat until browned.

2. Add broccoli florets and cauliflower rice to the skillet.

3. In a bowl, whisk together almond milk, grated Parmesan cheese, nutritional yeast, garlic powder, salt, and pepper.

4. Pour the sauce over the chicken and vegetables. Stir to combine.

5. Simmer for 15-20 minutes or until the broccoli is tender and the chicken is cooked through.

6. Serve hot.

Servings: 4

Nutritional Value (per serving):

- Calories: 320

- Protein: 30g

- Carbohydrates: 15g

- Fat: 15g

- Fiber: 5g

- Sugar: 3g

Cooking Time: 25 minutes

Guilt-Free Desserts

Ingredients:

- 1 cup mixed berries (strawberries, blueberries, raspberries)

- 1 cup Greek yogurt (unsweetened)

- 1 tablespoon chia seeds

- 1 teaspoon honey or stevia (optional)

- Fresh mint for garnish

Instructions:

1. In a bowl, mix Greek yogurt and chia seeds. Let it sit for 15 minutes.

2. In serving glasses, layer Greek yogurt mixture with mixed berries.

3. Repeat the layers.

4. Drizzle honey or add stevia if desired.

5. Garnish with fresh mint.

6. Refrigerate for at least 30 minutes before serving.

Servings: 2

Nutritional Value (per serving):

- Calories: 150

- Protein: 10g

- Carbohydrates: 15g

- Fat: 5g

- Fiber: 5g

- Sugar: 8g

Preparation Time: 15 minutes

2. Avocado Chocolate Mousse:

Ingredients:

- 2 ripe avocados

- 1/4 cup unsweetened cocoa powder

- 1/4 cup almond milk (unsweetened)

- 2 tablespoons maple syrup or stevia

- 1 teaspoon vanilla extract

- Pinch of salt

- Fresh berries for topping

Instructions:

1. In a blender, combine avocados, cocoa powder, almond milk, maple syrup (or stevia), vanilla extract, and a pinch of salt.

2. Blend until smooth and creamy.

3. Divide into serving bowls.

4. Refrigerate for at least 2 hours.

5. Top with fresh berries before serving.

Servings: 4

Nutritional Value (per serving):

- Calories: 180

- Protein: 3g

- Carbohydrates: 15g

- Fat: 14g

- Fiber: 7g

- Sugar: 5g

Preparation Time: 10 minutes

Ingredients:

- 1/4 cup chia seeds
- 1 cup coconut milk (unsweetened)
- 1 tablespoon shredded coconut (unsweetened)
- 1 teaspoon vanilla extract
- 1 tablespoon sliced almonds
- Berries for topping

Instructions:

1. In a bowl, mix chia seeds, coconut milk, shredded coconut, and vanilla extract.
2. Let it sit in the refrigerator for at least 4 hours or overnight.
3. Stir well before serving.
4. Top with sliced almonds and berries.

Servings: 2

Nutritional Value (per serving): Calories: 200, Protein: 5g, Carbohydrates: 15g, Fat: 15g, Fiber: 8g, Sugar: 2g

Preparation Time: 5 minutes (plus chilling time)

4. Baked Apples with Cinnamon:

Ingredients:

- 2 apples, cored and sliced
- 1 teaspoon cinnamon
- 1 tablespoon chopped walnuts (optional)
- 1 tablespoon honey or stevia
- Greek yogurt for serving

Instructions:

1. Preheat the oven to 375°F (190°C).
2. In a bowl, toss apple slices with cinnamon and chopped walnuts.
3. Arrange the apples in a baking dish.
4. Drizzle with honey or sprinkle with stevia.
5. Bake for 20-25 minutes or until apples are tender.
6. Serve with a dollop of Greek yogurt.

Servings: 2

Nutritional Value (per serving): Calories: 120, Protein: 2g, Carbohydrates: 25g, Fat: 3g, Fiber: 5g, Sugar: 18g

Cooking Time: 25 minutes

Ingredients:

- 1 cup almond flour
- 1/2 cup vanilla protein powder (unsweetened)
- 1/4 cup coconut flour
- 1 teaspoon baking powder
- 1/2 teaspoon cinnamon
- 1/4 teaspoon nutmeg
- 1/4 teaspoon salt
- 1/2 cup canned pumpkin
- 1/4 cup almond milk (unsweetened)
- 2 tablespoons coconut oil, melted
- 2 tablespoons maple syrup or stevia
- 1 teaspoon vanilla extract
- Chopped pecans for topping

Instructions:

1. Preheat the oven to 350°F (175°C). Line a muffin tin with paper liners.

2. In a bowl, whisk together almond flour, protein powder, coconut flour, baking powder, cinnamon, nutmeg, and salt.

3. In another bowl, mix canned pumpkin, almond milk, melted coconut oil, maple syrup (or stevia), and vanilla extract.

4. Combine wet and dry ingredients until well combined.

5. Spoon the batter into muffin cups.

6. Top each muffin with chopped pecans.

7. Bake for 20-25 minutes or until a toothpick comes out clean.

Servings: 6

Nutritional Value (per serving):

- Calories: 180

- Protein: 10g

- Carbohydrates: 10g

- Fat: 12g

- Fiber: 4g

- Sugar: 4g

Cooking Time: 25 minutes

Ingredients:

- 1 cup almond flour
- 1/2 cup vanilla protein powder (unsweetened)
- 1/4 cup coconut flour
- Zest and juice of 1 lemon
- 1/4 cup almond butter
- 1/4 cup coconut oil, melted
- 2 tablespoons maple syrup or stevia
- 1 teaspoon vanilla extract
- 1 tablespoon poppy seeds

Instructions:

1. Line a baking dish with parchment paper.
2. In a bowl, combine almond flour, protein powder, coconut flour, lemon zest, and poppy seeds.
3. In another bowl, mix almond butter, melted coconut oil, maple syrup (or stevia), lemon juice, and vanilla extract.

4. Combine wet and dry ingredients until a dough forms.

5. Press the dough into the baking dish.

6. Refrigerate for at least 2 hours before cutting into bars.

Servings: 8

Nutritional Value (per serving):

- Calories: 150

- Protein: 8g

- Carbohydrates: 8g

- Fat: 10g

- Fiber: 3g

- Sugar: 3g

Preparation Time: 15 minutes (plus chilling time)

These guilt-free desserts are designed to be bariatric-friendly and suitable for individuals managing diabetes, heart disease, kidney health, and weight loss.

Chapter 6:

Overcoming Challenges and Celebrating Success

Dealing with Food Intolerances

Dealing with food intolerances is a crucial aspect of maintaining a healthy and balanced diet, especially for individuals who have undergone gastric sleeve surgery. Food intolerances occur when the digestive system has difficulty processing certain foods, leading to various uncomfortable symptoms. Here's a comprehensive guide on how to handle food intolerances:

1. Identify Trigger Foods:

- Keep a detailed food diary to track what you eat and any symptoms you experience.

- Note patterns of discomfort or adverse reactions to specific foods.

2. Consult with Healthcare Professionals:

- Work closely with your healthcare team, including your surgeon, nutritionist, and other relevant specialists.

- Discuss any symptoms or concerns related to food intolerances during follow-up appointments.

3. Recognize Common Intolerances:

- Be aware of common food intolerances, such as lactose, gluten, and certain artificial additives.

- Consider allergy testing or specialized diagnostic tests to pinpoint specific intolerances.

4. Gradual Reintroduction:

- If a particular food is suspected to cause intolerance, consider reintroducing it gradually in small amounts.

- Monitor your body's response and adjust intake based on tolerance levels.

5. Choose Alternatives:

- Opt for alternative ingredients that are well-tolerated and provide similar nutritional benefits.

- Explore gluten-free, lactose-free, or other suitable substitutes for problematic foods.

6. Practice Mindful Eating:

- Eat slowly and pay attention to your body's signals.

- Note any discomfort or adverse reactions during and after meals.

7. Read Food Labels:

- Become adept at reading food labels to identify potential triggers.

- Look for hidden ingredients that may contribute to intolerance symptoms.

8. Stay Hydrated:

- Adequate hydration is essential for digestive health.

- Water can help alleviate symptoms and support the overall digestive process.

9. Support Digestive Health:

- Include foods rich in probiotics, such as yogurt with live cultures or fermented foods, to promote a healthy gut microbiome.

- Consider digestive enzyme supplements to aid in the breakdown of certain foods.

10. Monitor Nutrient Levels:

- Regularly check nutrient levels through blood tests to identify deficiencies.

- Adjust your diet or supplement regimen as necessary to maintain optimal nutritional status.

11. Emotional Well-being:

- Recognize the emotional impact of food intolerances and seek support if needed.

- Emotional well-being is crucial for maintaining a positive relationship with food and overall health.

Remember, managing food intolerances is a personalized journey, and it's essential to work closely with healthcare professionals to tailor strategies to your specific needs.

Regular communication with your healthcare team will help address any challenges and ensure your nutritional plan aligns with your post-surgery requirements.

Staying Motivated on Your Journey

Staying motivated on your journey, especially after undergoing gastric sleeve surgery, is vital for achieving long-term success in maintaining a healthy lifestyle. Here are some strategies to help you stay motivated:

1. Set Realistic Goals:

- Establish clear, achievable goals that align with your overall health and well-being.

- Break down larger goals into smaller, manageable steps to track progress more effectively.

2. Celebrate Achievements:

- Acknowledge and celebrate both big and small accomplishments.

- Reward yourself for reaching milestones, whether it's fitting into a smaller clothing size or consistently meeting exercise targets.

3. Create a Support System:

- Surround yourself with a supportive network of friends, family, and fellow individuals who understand and encourage your journey.

- Share your goals with them to receive positive reinforcement.

4. Track Your Progress:

- Keep a record of your achievements, changes in health, and positive feedback from healthcare professionals.

- Regularly review your progress to stay motivated and reinforce the positive impact of your efforts.

5. Embrace Variety:

- Introduce variety into your exercise routine and meal plans to prevent boredom.

- Experiment with new recipes, activities, or fitness classes to keep things interesting.

6. Focus on Non-Scale Victories:

- Recognize achievements beyond the scale, such as improved energy levels, enhanced mood, or better sleep quality.

- Shift the focus from just weight loss to overall well-being.

7. Visualize Success:

- Create a mental image of your desired outcome and visualize the positive impact your efforts will have on your life.

- Use visualization techniques to reinforce your commitment and motivation.

8. Establish Routine:

- Develop a consistent daily routine that includes healthy habits.

- Routines can create stability and make it easier to incorporate positive behaviors into your lifestyle.

9. Stay Educated:

- Continuously educate yourself about nutrition, fitness, and overall health.

- Understanding the benefits of your choices can reinforce motivation and commitment.

10. Be Kind to Yourself:

- Accept that setbacks may occur, and view them as opportunities to learn and adjust.

- Practice self-compassion and avoid being overly critical. Remember that it's a journey, not a race.

11. Join a Community:

- Connect with others who share similar goals by joining support groups, online forums, or fitness classes.

- Sharing experiences and challenges can provide motivation and a sense of camaraderie.

12. Reassess and Adjust Goals:

- Regularly reassess your goals and adjust them based on changing circumstances or priorities.

- Ensure that your goals remain relevant and achievable.

Remember that maintaining motivation is an ongoing process. By incorporating these strategies into your daily life, you can create a positive and sustainable mindset that supports your journey to improved health and well-being.

CONCLUSION

In conclusion, this Gastric Sleeve Bariatric Cookbook serves not just as a collection of nutritious recipes but as a comprehensive guide to support your journey towards a healthier and more fulfilling life after gastric sleeve surgery. By emphasizing the importance of tailored nutrition, mindful eating, and a positive mindset, this cookbook aims to empower you to make informed choices that contribute to sustained well-being.

As you embark on this transformative culinary adventure, remember that each recipe is crafted with your post-surgery nutritional needs in mind. From the basics of gastric sleeve nutrition to the delightful and bariatric-friendly breakfasts, lunches, dinners, and guilt-free desserts, these recipes are designed to nourish your body while satisfying your taste buds.

Your path to optimal health is not just about the food on your plate but also about embracing a lifestyle that encourages self-care, self-discovery, and resilience. This cookbook is a companion on your journey, providing practical tips, insights, and flavorful creations that make adopting a bariatric-friendly diet an enjoyable and sustainable choice.

So, let each meal be a celebration of your commitment to health, and let each page of this cookbook be a step towards a revitalized and vibrant you. Your journey is unique, and this cookbook is here to inspire and guide you every step of the way. Remember, the most meaningful change comes from within, and by choosing the path of nourishment, you are not just transforming your diet – you are embracing a life filled with vitality, balance, and lasting well-being. Let the joy of these recipes be your constant motivation, encouraging you to savor the flavors of health and happiness on your extraordinary journey.

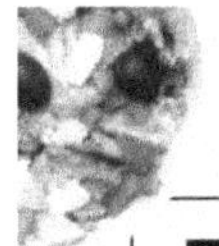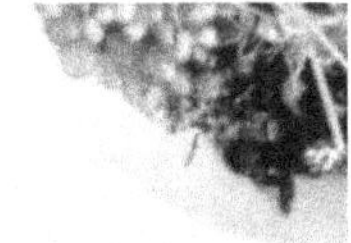

MEAL PLANNER

DATE:

	BREAKFAST	LUNCH	DINNER	SHOPPING LIST
MON				
TUES				
WED				
THURS				
FRI				
SAT				
SUN				

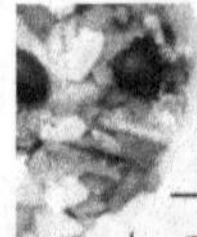
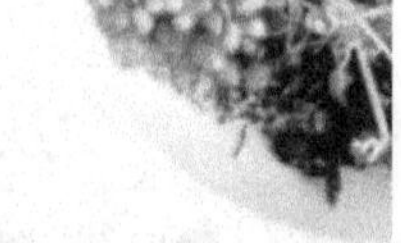

MEAL PLANNER

DATE:

	BREAKFAST	LUNCH	DINNER	SHOPPING LIST
MON				
TUES				
WED				
THURS				
FRI				
SAT				
SUN				

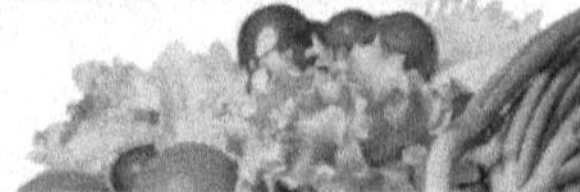

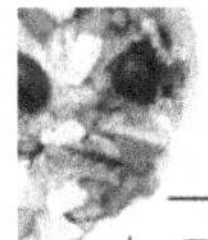
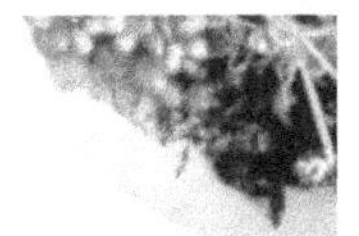

MEAL PLANNER

DATE:

	BREAKFAST	LUNCH	DINNER	SHOPPING LIST
MON				
TUES				
WED				
THURS				
FRI				
SAT				
SUN				

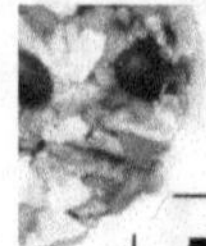

MEAL PLANNER

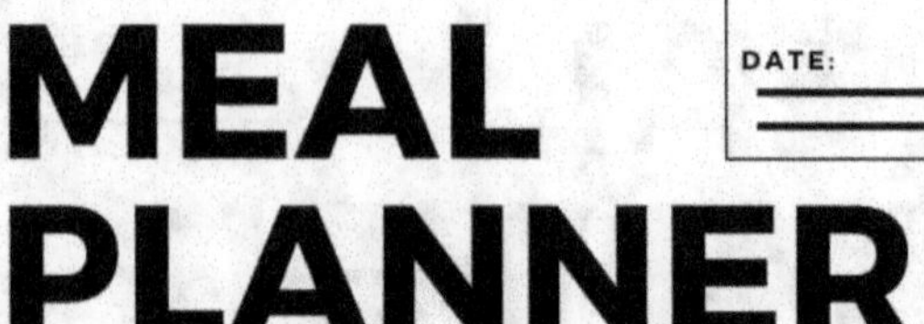

DATE:

	BREAKFAST	LUNCH	DINNER	SHOPPING LIST
MON				
TUES				
WED				
THURS				
FRI				
SAT				
SUN				

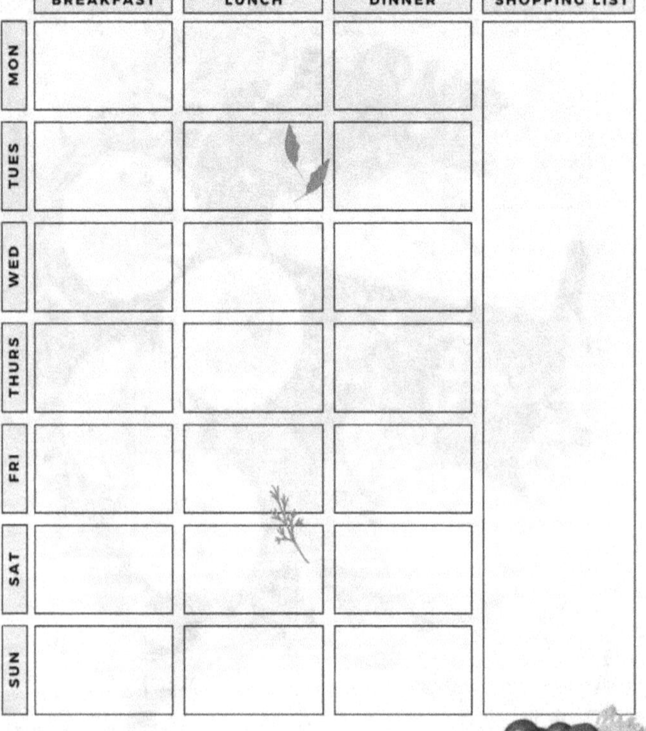

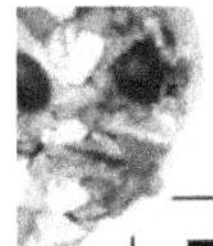
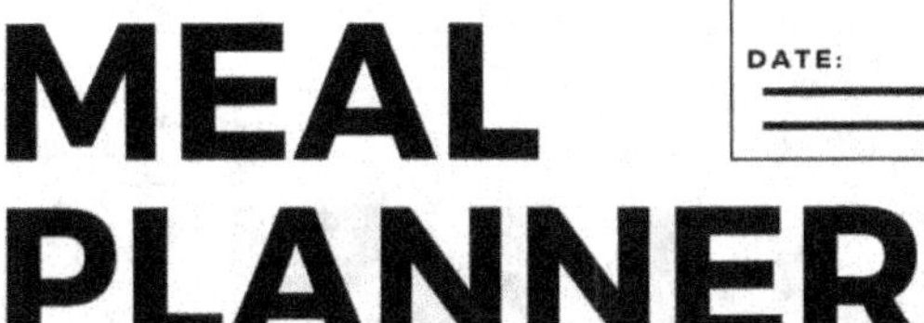

MEAL PLANNER

DATE: ___________

	BREAKFAST	LUNCH	DINNER	SHOPPING LIST
MON				
TUES				
WED				
THURS				
FRI				
SAT				
SUN				

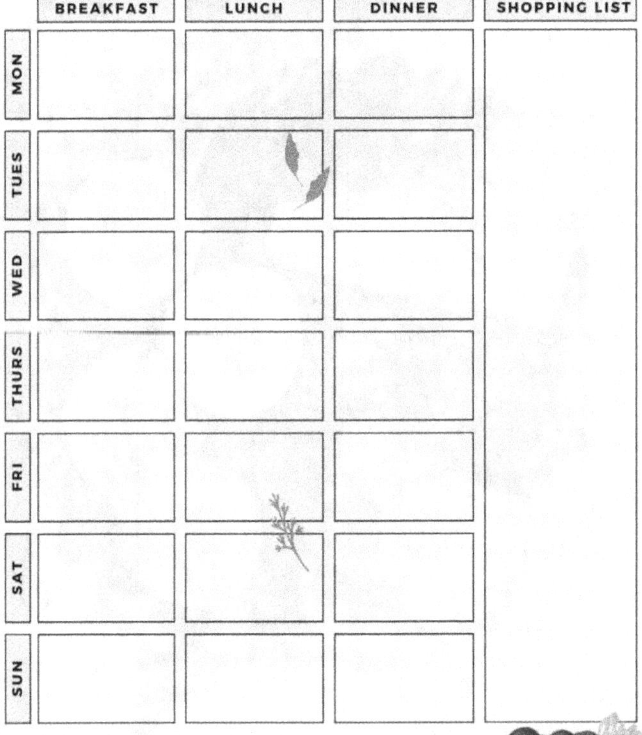

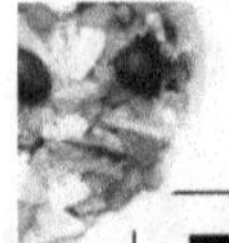

MEAL PLANNER

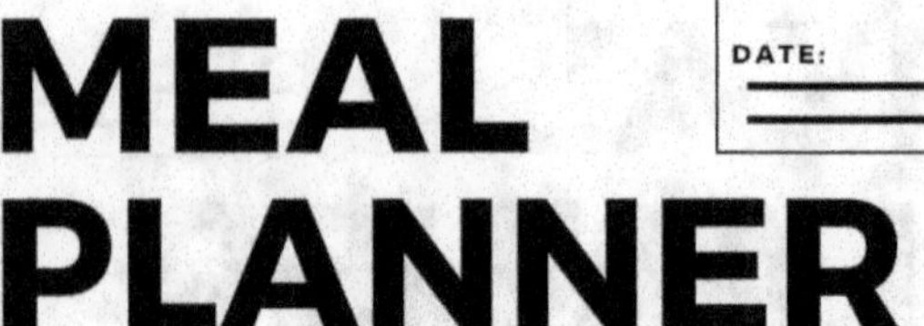

DATE:

	BREAKFAST	LUNCH	DINNER	SHOPPING LIST
MON				
TUES				
WED				
THURS				
FRI				
SAT				
SUN				

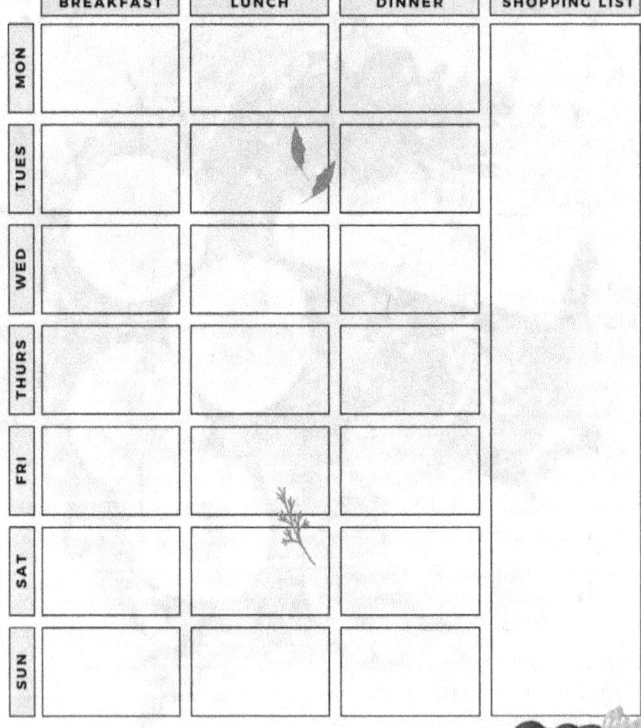

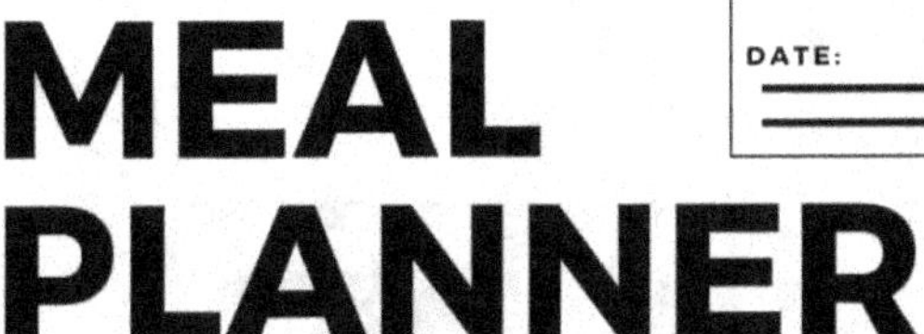

MEAL PLANNER

DATE: ___________

	BREAKFAST	LUNCH	DINNER	SHOPPING LIST
MON				
TUES				
WED				
THURS				
FRI				
SAT				
SUN				

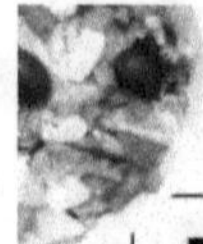
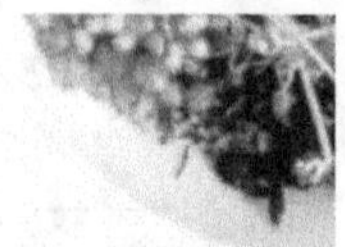

MEAL PLANNER

DATE: ___________

	BREAKFAST	LUNCH	DINNER	SHOPPING LIST
MON				
TUES				
WED				
THURS				
FRI				
SAT				
SUN				

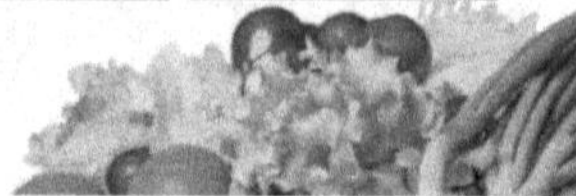

MEAL PLANNER

DATE:

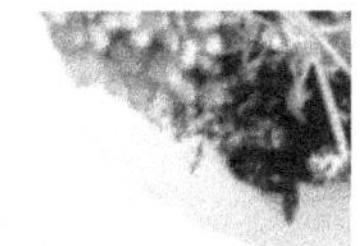

	BREAKFAST	LUNCH	DINNER	SHOPPING LIST
MON				
TUES				
WED				
THURS				
FRI				
SAT				
SUN				

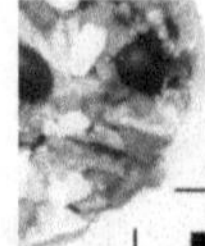
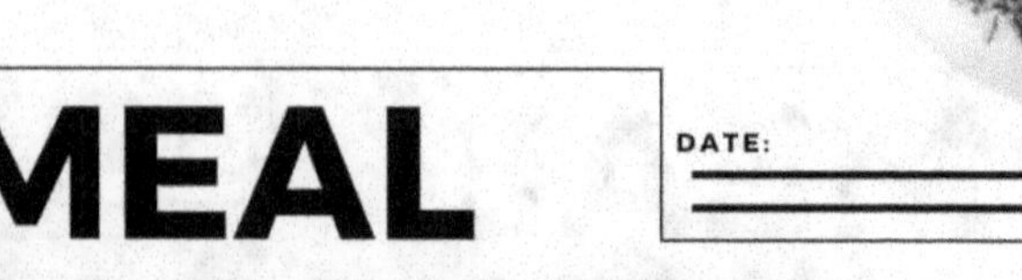

MEAL PLANNER

DATE:

	BREAKFAST	LUNCH	DINNER	SHOPPING LIST
MON				
TUES				
WED				
THURS				
FRI				
SAT				
SUN				

MEAL PLANNER

DATE:

	BREAKFAST	LUNCH	DINNER	SHOPPING LIST
MON				
TUES				
WED				
THURS				
FRI				
SAT				
SUN				

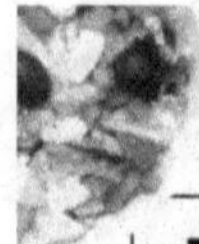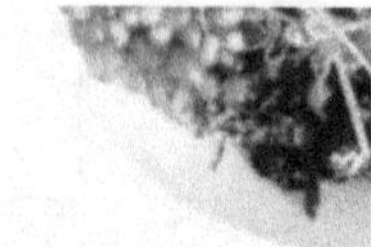

MEAL PLANNER

DATE:

	BREAKFAST	LUNCH	DINNER	SHOPPING LIST
MON				
TUES				
WED				
THURS				
FRI				
SAT				
SUN				

MEAL PLANNER

DATE:

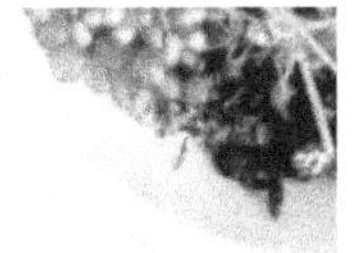

	BREAKFAST	LUNCH	DINNER	SHOPPING LIST
MON				
TUES				
WED				
THURS				
FRI				
SAT				
SUN				

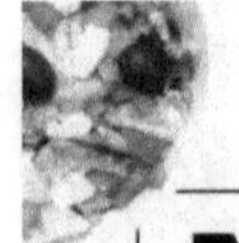

MEAL PLANNER

DATE:

	BREAKFAST	LUNCH	DINNER	SHOPPING LIST
MON				
TUES				
WED				
THURS				
FRI				
SAT				
SUN				

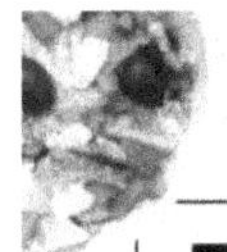

MEAL PLANNER

DATE:

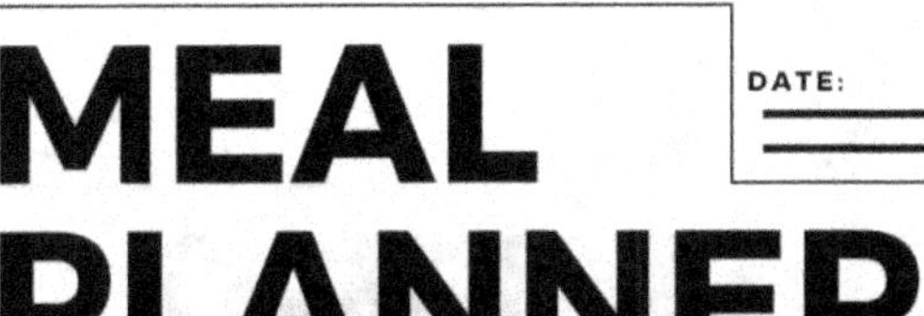

	BREAKFAST	LUNCH	DINNER	SHOPPING LIST
MON				
TUES				
WED				
THURS				
FRI				
SAT				
SUN				

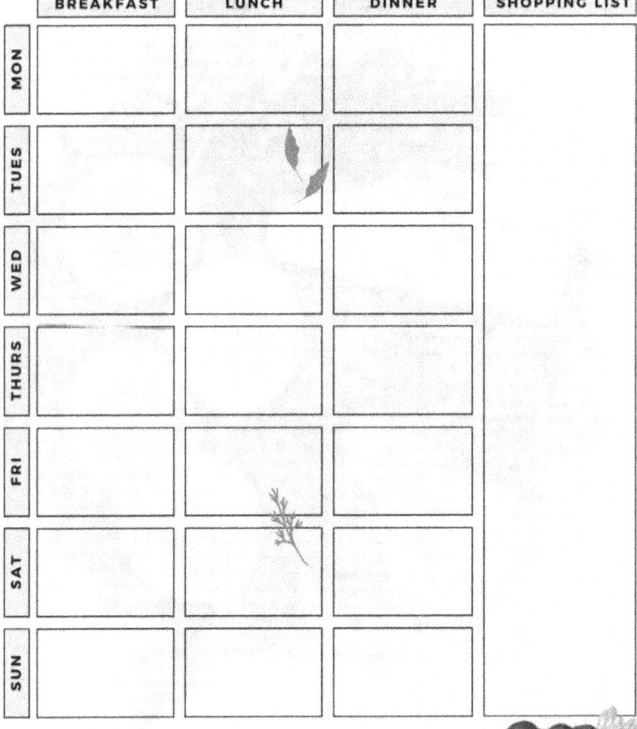

MEAL PLANNER

DATE:

	BREAKFAST	LUNCH	DINNER	SHOPPING LIST
MON				
TUES				
WED				
THURS				
FRI				
SAT				
SUN				

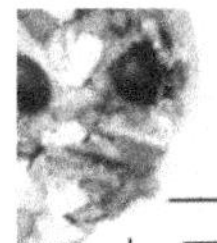

MEAL PLANNER

DATE:

	BREAKFAST	LUNCH	DINNER	SHOPPING LIST
MON				
TUES				
WED				
THURS				
FRI				
SAT				
SUN				

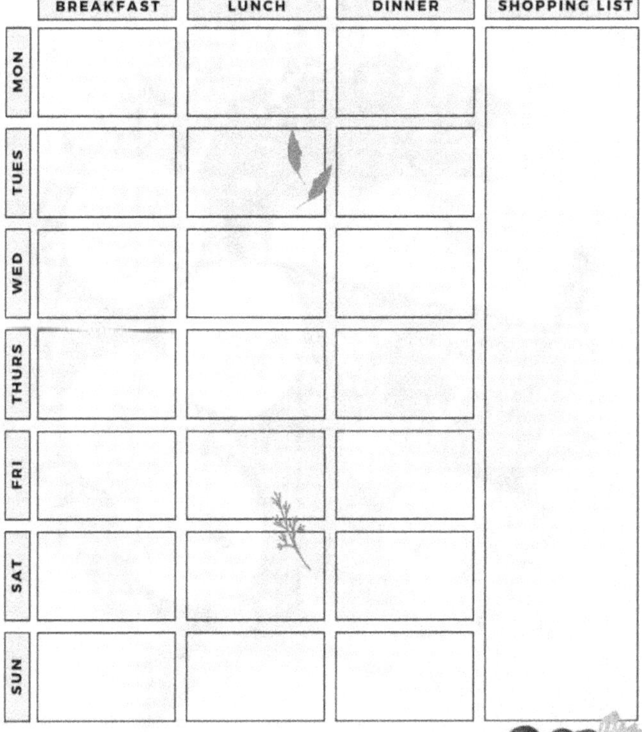

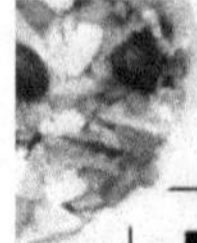

MEAL PLANNER

DATE: ___________

	BREAKFAST	LUNCH	DINNER	SHOPPING LIST
MON				
TUES				
WED				
THURS				
FRI				
SAT				
SUN				

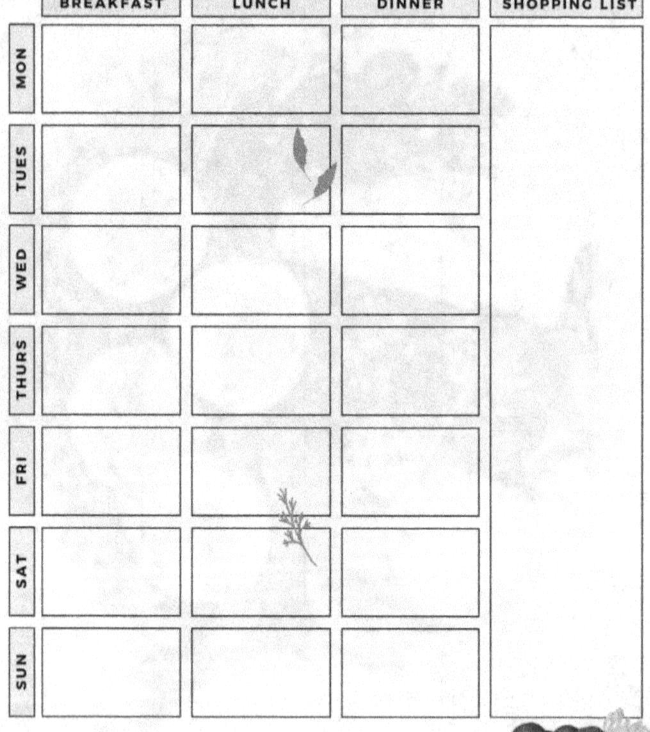

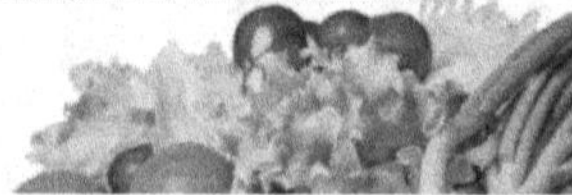

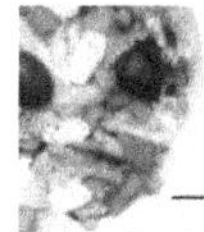

MEAL PLANNER

DATE:

	BREAKFAST	LUNCH	DINNER	SHOPPING LIST
MON				
TUES				
WED				
THURS				
FRI				
SAT				
SUN				

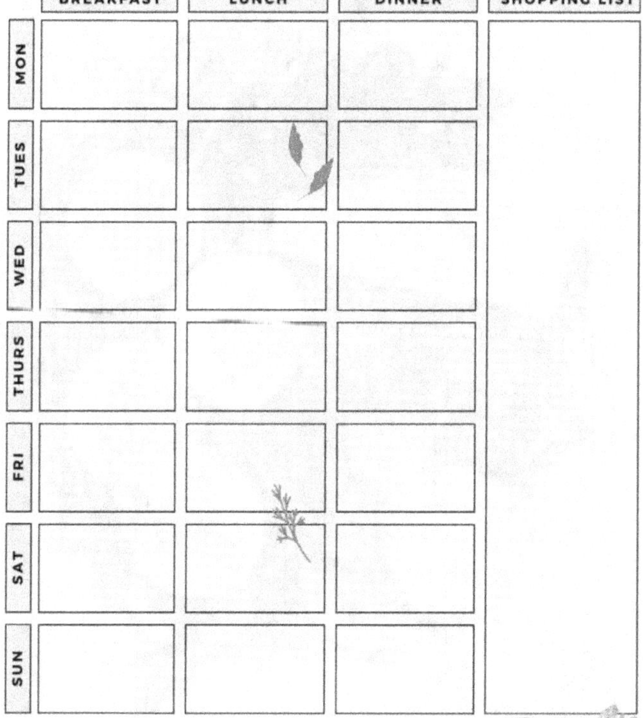

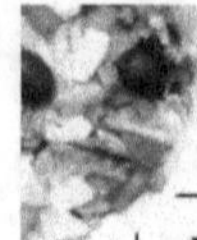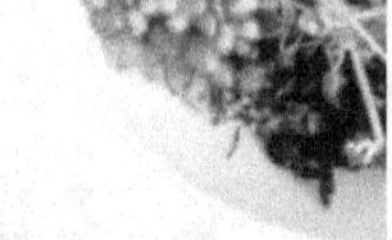

MEAL PLANNER

DATE:

	BREAKFAST	LUNCH	DINNER	SHOPPING LIST
MON				
TUES				
WED				
THURS				
FRI				
SAT				
SUN				

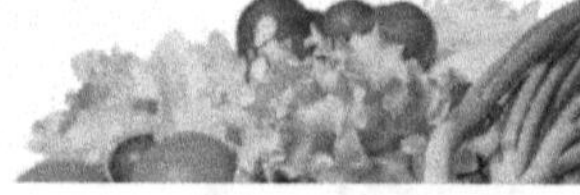